MOTOR
CONTROL

MOTOR CONTROL

Edited by

G. N. Gantchev

B. Dimitrov

and

P. Gatev

Institute of Physiology
Bulgarian Academy of Sciences
Sofia, Bulgaria

PLENUM PRESS • NEW YORK AND LONDON

Library of Congress Cataloging in Publication Data

International Symposium on Motor Control (5th: 1985: Varna, Bulgaria)
    Motor control.

    "Proceedings of the Fifth International Symposium on Motor Control, held
June 10–15, 1985, in Varna, Bulgaria"—T.p. verso.
    Includes bibliographies and index.
    1. Neuromuscular transmission—Congresses. 2. Sensory-motor integration—
Congresses. 3. Afferent pathways—Congresses. 4. Locomotion—Regulation—
Congresses. I. Gantchev, G. N. II. Dimitrov, B. III. Gatev, P. IV. Title. [DNLM:
1. Motor Activity—congresses. 2. Movement—congresses. 3. Nervous System—
physiology—congresses. 4. Posture—congresses. W3 IN91985 5th 1985m / WE
103 I601 1985m]
QP369.5.I58   1985   599′.01852   87-2326
ISBN 978-1-4615-7510-8   ISBN 978-1-4615-7508-5 (eBook)
DOI 10.1007/978-1-4615-7508-5

Proceedings of the Fifth International Symposium on Motor Control,
held June 10–15, 1985, in Varna, Bulgaria

© 1987 Plenum Press, New York
Softcover reprint of the hardcover 1st edition 1987

A Division of Plenum Publishing Corporation
233 Spring Street, New York, N.Y. 10013

PREFACE

This book encompasses part of the papers presented at the Fifth International Symposium on Motor Control held in Varna, Bulgaria from 10 to 14 June 1985. The Motor Control Symposia organized in Bulgaria became tradition following the successful initiation of Professor Gydikov and his collaborators of the previous four meetings (Sofia, 1969, Varna, 1972, Albena, 1976, Varna, 1981). More than 140 scientists participated in the last Symposium, 40 from East Europe, 15 from West Europe, 15 from USA and Canada. These Symposia established an opportunity for encounter of prominent scientists from all over the world, representatives of different schools and mainstreams. The participation of R. Granit, W. R. Ashby, B. C. Matthews, V. S. Gurfinkel, E. V. Evarts etc., is to be mentioned.

The main topics of the Symposium included: 1) Motor Unit Activity; 2) Reflex Control of Movements; 3) Central Control of Movements; 4) Posture Control; 5) Locomotion; 6) Arm Movement; 7) Motor Control Models. 43 oral presentations and 103 posters were reported, 36 of them being presented in this volume.

The presented papers deal with the complex mechanisms of movement and posture control, investigations of considerable interest in recent years. This interest was prompted by the huge biological importance of the motor activity as a most common mechanism of adaptation to the environment. Motor activity is also inadvertently involved in various fields of human practice: occupational activities, including extreme conditions, motor handicaps, sports, bioprosthetic devices, bionics, robotics etc.

The problem of central mechanisms of movement and postural regulation was enlightened by new data concerning the role of various brain structures and certain psychophysiological processes in the organization of the motor activity. Some neurophysiological data concern, more or less directly, the question of voluntary control of movements and posture - a problem that occupies central position in the motor control versatility. The invited lecture of Dr Edward Evarts, unfortunately no longer with us, was dedicated to the problem of the neurophysiological mechanisms of the central control of movements. An obituary, prepared with the collaboration of Jerome Sanes from NINCDS at NIH, Bethesda, appears in this book with our deepest reverence to that eminent man and scientist. Dr Evarts was a great friend of the physiologists from Eastern Europe and, especially, Bulgaria. Dr G. N. Gantchev, Head of the Department of Motor Control at the Institute of Physiology, Bulgarian Academy of Sciences worked for some time in the Laboratory of Neurophysiology in Bethesda. Dr Evarts visited the Institute of Physiology in Bulgaria in 1980 and was a guest of honor at the Symposium. He also was delegated the mission of further extending collaboration in the field of neuroscience between National Academy of Sciences in USA and Bulgarian Academy of Sciences.

The problem of sensory control of movements posture and locomotion stands in relevant position. The role of different sensory inputs for the reflex and central regulation of movements and posture, their relationship and integration at different functional levels was discussed.

New data were presented regarding the peripheral control of movements and posture; activity of alpha-motoneurones and Motor Unit Activity in phasic movements and gait with different patterns of muscular activity; and the functional differentiation of MUs.

Parallel to the studies of different links in the system for control of movements and posture, investigations involving certain mechanisms at system level emerged. They comprise the investigation of some biomechanical features of voluntary movements and locomotion. This approach to the study of motor activity nowadays acquired immense importance due to the fact that data about biomechanical investigation at the system output level and about neurophysiological action of its separate levels are being synthesized. Some of the studies dealing with models of motor regulation presented examples of this multifarious state of the art.

A characteristic feature in the recent exploration of motor activity is the ever increasing number of human studies. It is demonstrated in two thirds of the works presented in this book. This scientific venue has the obvious advantage of prompt prospects for application into practice. Some papers were devoted to the clinical neurophysiology studying mechanisms of regulation in motor disturbances: a fruitful approach assisting the treatment of neurological patients.

The multitude of the presented papers assessing different neurophysiological, psychophysiological and biomechanical aspects of the motor control in normal and pathological conditions creates opportunity for estimation of the data in their complex interrelationships in the regulation system as a whole, for synthesis of the various fragments, for begetting of new ideas and widening of the current knowledge. This standpoint was proved also during the discussions at the Symposium and we do hope that the reader will appreciate the book from this viewpoint as well.

Unfortunately, a considerable amount of papers related to important problems of motor control did not find place in this book hindered by either volume restrictions or presentation elsewhere.

Our thanks are going to Plenum Publishing Corporation Ltd., for their valuable help and encouragement while preparing this book, an extension of our collaboration since the first Motor Control volume from 1973, comprising papers presented at the Second Symposium of Motor Control. We thank too all contributors and participants in the Symposium as well.

G. N. Gantchev
Editor

CONTENTS

Edward Vaughn Evarts   xi

SECTION I.   MOTOR UNIT ACTIVITY

The Pattern-Related Modifications of Contractile Response
    of Human Skeletal Muscle
    V. S. Gurfinkel and Yu. S. Levik   3

Motor Unit Discharges in Interosseus Dorsalis Primus Muscle
    during Voluntary Movements
    D. Kosarov, A. Gydikov, and A. Kossev   7

The Use of Low and High Threshold Units during Voluntary
    Contraction and Locomotion
    L. Grimby   13

Measurement and Characteristics of Recurrent IPSPs Produced
    by Stimulation of Single Motor Axons
    T. M. Hamm, C.-S. Yuan, S.-I. Sasaki, and D. G. Stuart   19

Application of Cross-Sectional Single-Fiber Microchemistry
    to the Study of Motor-Unit Fatigability
    P. M. Nemeth, T. M. Hamm, D. A. Gordon, R. M. Reinking,
    and D. G. Stuart   23

SECTION II.   REFLEX CONTROL OF MOVEMENTS

Development of Cutaneous Reflexes in the Upper Limb during
    Man Ontogenesis
    V. Gatev, M. Stefanova-Uzunova, and L. Stamatova   31

M2-A Long Latency Spinal Reflex Due to Skin Afferents in Man
    M. Shahani, O. C. J. Lippold, K. Darton, and U. Shahani   37

Factors which Modify the Short and Long Latency Components
    of the Stretch Reflex in the Human Forearm
    R. G. Lee, R. Hayashi, and W. Becker   43

Changes in Stretch Responses due to Hypotonia
    A. Struppler, H. Riescher, and L. Gerilovsky   51

Presynaptic Inhibition and Disinhibition of Monosynaptic
    Reflex in Man
    R. Person and G. Kozhina   59

The Differentiation of Golgi Tendon Organs in the Rat Hind
    Limb Muscles after Neonatal De-efferentation
    T. Soukup and J. Zelená   63

SECTION III. CENTRAL CONTROL OF MOVEMENTS

Trigeminal Afferents to the Fastigial n. and Paleocerebellar
    Modulation of Hypoglossal Motoneurons: Neuroanatomical
    and Electrophysiological Study Suggesting a Trans-
    cerebellar Loop for Tongue Muscle Activity Regulation
    A. Bava, F. Fabbro, S. Mininel-Conte, G. Leanza, A. Russo,
    and S. Stanzani   69

EMG and Hippocampal EEG Activities during Spontaneous and
    Elicited Movements in the Rat
    R. Korczyński, S. Kasicki, and U. Borecka   75

Higher Disturbances of Movement in Monkeys (macaca fascicularis)
    U. Halsband   79

Characteristics of Dentate Neuronal Discharge in a Simple
    and a Choice Reaction Time Task in the Monkey
    C. E. Chapman and Y. Lamarre   87

Movement Related Brain Potentials in Sustained Isometric
    Voluntary Contraction
    B. Dimitrov, G. N. Gantchev, and D. Popivanov   93

Are Self-Paced Repetitive Fatiguing Hand Contractions Accompanied
    by Changes in Movement-Related Brain Potentials?
    G. Freude, P. Ullsperger, and M. Pietschmann   99

Effects of Antagonist Activation on Sensations of Muscle Force
    L. Jones and I. Hunter   105

Initiation of Electromyographic Activity in Fast Forward Arm
    Elevation
    P. Gatev, G. N. Gantchev, R. Koedjikova, and B. Dimitrov   111

SECTION IV. POSTURE CONTROL

Bulbar Reticular Unit Activity Relating to Posture and Skilled
    Forelimb Movement in Rats
    M. Šaling, J. Kundrát, and P. Duda   119

Putative Neurophysiological and Neurochemical Mechanisms Under-
    lying Striatal Control of Postural Adjustment in Dogs
    K. B. Shapovalova and I. V. Yakunin   123

Role of the Visual Feedback for Stabilization of Vertical Human
    Posture during Induced Body Oscillations
    G. N. Gantchev, P. Gatev, N. Tankov, N. Draganova, S. Dunev
    and D. Popivanov   129
Afferent Control of Posture and Gait
    J. Quintern, W. Berger, and V. Dietz   135

Facilitation of Vestibulo-Motor Response by Voluntary Movements
    in Man
    B. N. Smetanin, V. Ju. Shlikov, and M. P. Kudinova   141

Evaluation of Mechanisms of Postural Regulation by Means of
    Time Series Analysis
    D. Bräuer and H. Seidel   145

The Effect of Support Unloading on Characteristics of Motor
    Control Systems Activity
    I. B. Kozlovskaya, I. F. Aslanova, and A. V. Kirenskaya   149

SECTION V.   LOCOMOTION

Activity of Ventral Spinocerebellar Tract Neurons
    Chronically Recorded in the Spinal Cord of Awake,
    Freely Moving Cats
    C. L. Cleland and J. A. Hoffer   155

Activity Patterns of Identified Alpha Motoneurons to Cat Anterior
    Thigh Muscles during Normal Walking and Flexor Reflexes
    G. E. Loeb, J. A. Hoffer, N. Sugano, W. B. Marks,
    M. J. O'Donovan, and G. A. Pratt   159

Antidromic Discharges of Primary Afferents during Locomotion
    R. Dubuc, J.-M. Cabelguen, and S. Rossignol   165

Responses of the Forelimb to Perturbations Applied during the
    Swing Phase of the Step Cycle
    T. Drew and S. Rossignol   171

Comparative Analysis of the Kinematical Characteristics of
    Man's Walking in the Ontogeny
    E. N. Artemjeva and V. V. Smolyaninov   177

SECTION VI.   MOTOR CONTROL MODELS

A Model for One-Joint Motor Control in Man
    R. M. Abdusamatov, S. V. Adamovich, and A. G. Feldman   183

System Identification in Motor Control: Time-Varying
    Techniques
    I. Hunter and R. Kearney   189

Workspace Effect in Arm Movement Kinematics Derived by
    Joint Interpolation
    J. M. Hollerbach, S. P. Moore, and C. G. Atkeson   197

Kinematic Form of Limb and Speech Movements
    D. J. Ostry, J. D. Cooke, and K. G. Munhall   209

Synergetics at Motoneuron Level
    St. Baykushev   215

Index   219

EDWARD VAUGHN EVARTS

Bethesda, Maryland
12 November 1985

Edward Vaughn Evarts died on the morning of 2 July 1985 from a heart attack at the age of 59. He had just returned to Bethesda earlier than planned, and seemingly healthy, from a trip to Eastern Europe and to Finland; the native country of his wife Ritva. On this trip, the last of many to Eastern Europe, Ed participated in an international symposium on Motor Control; this book represents the record of that meeting. Although the content of his address to the meeting was on brain neuronal activity and movement, discussions at the symposium further stimulated Ed's interest in human motor control. Forthwith he conceived a series of experiments to study the relationships between voluntary movement and cerebral events in humans. These studies, due to begin soon after the arrival to the Laboratory of Neurophysiology of a colleague from Bulgaria, were a major topic of conversation in the laboratory on the morning of Ed's death and a reason for his early return. Although this work represented a departure for Ed from previous research methods and questions, it demonstrated a willingness to pursue new ideas and inject new techniques into his search to understand brain function.

In between medical training at Harvard University and a medical residency at the Payne Whitney Clinic in New York and a neurology fellowship at the National Hospital for Nervous Diseases in London, Ed began his research career at the Yerkes Primate Research Center, then located in Orange Park, Florida, under the direction of Karl Lashley. Ed's studies at Yerkes were concerned with the behavioral effects of ablation of auditory and nonprimary visual cortex in monkeys. Perhaps it was Lashley's influence that imbued Ed with the often stated goal of investigating questions relating to whole brain function and not simply with questions designed to provide small increments in knowledge about how the brain worked.

In 1953, Ed began a 32 year association with the National Institute of Mental Health that culminated in 1970 with his position as Chief of the Laboratory of Neurophysiology. At first Ed studied the effects of psychoactive drugs on the brain, but soon devoted his attention to understanding brain physiology by recording responses in the primary visual pathways to electrical and photic stimulation. Later on he investigated spontaneous activity in the visual cortex during sleep and waking. These studies led directly to those on the motor cortex of the monkey for which Ed's contribution to neurobiology are best known. He is generally credited with making the critical developments in the method of chronic single unit recording, first originated by Jasper and Hubel, so that the method became a practical means of neurophysiological investigation. That countless neurophysiologists now employ this method to evaluate the activity of

neurons in awake animals is testament enough to Ed's contribution to neurobiology. However, Ed was not satisfied merely with technological inno-
vation. His seminal studies on the discharge properties of physiologically
identified neurons in the motor cortex of monkeys that performed voluntary
movements stand as important contributions not only to motor control research but also to integrative neurophysiologists as paradigms. Ed's
interests extended to many aspects of neurobiology; a reflection of that
was direct participation in studies of human motor control in both normal
subjects and those with neurological disorders and support of research
within the Laboratory of Neurophysiology into the physiological, anatomical
and chemical organization of the cerebral cortex, basal ganglia, thalamus
and cerebellum. All of these interests were well integrated as exemplified
by coordinated studies which evaluated the details of human movements or
neural responses in the motor cortex of monkeys in similar behavioral
tasks.

In addition to maintaining an active research and training program
which has produced several prominent neurobiologists, Ed contributed to the
worldwide development of neuroscience. A litany of his contributions could
not do justice to their collective impact but a few are nevertheless
remarkable. His trips to Eastern Europe were notable in that he communi-
cated the current state of neurophysiology to scientists there. Ed had a
major influence on the development of behavioral neurophysiology in Japan
due to a six month visit there in 1969 helping to establish a neurophysiology laboratory in Kyoto and the stream of young Japanese physiologists that visited Bethesda over the years. He was the current chairman
of the Neurobiology Section of the National Academy of Sciences, presiding
over a record number of inductees into that section of the Academy. Ed was
involved in the creation of the Society for Neuroscience and served as the
Society's President in 1974-1975 and as an Editor of the Neural Systems
Section of the Journal of Neuroscience from the inception of the journal.
Other editorial contributions were as Chief Editor for the Journal of
Neurophysiology from 1974-1977 and as a current member of the editorial
board for Trends in Neuroscience, Experimental Brain Research and the
Journal of Motor Behavior. An important contribution that Ed made to
neuroscience that may be unrecognized was his participation on many review
committees that ultimately awarded funds and prizes for neuroscience
research; most prominent among these were duties for the McKnight
Foundation and for the Albert Lasker Medical Research Awards. Ed's scientific contributions to research were acknowledged by several awards from
the United States Department of Health and Human Services, by peer-elected
memberships to the United States' National Academy of Sciences and the
Institute of Medicine and by the cherished Karl S. Lashley Award of the
American Philosophical Society.

Ed's death came as a great blow to all of us who knew him and
especially to those who had worked with and learned much from him in the
Laboratory of Neurophysiology. In a sense, the greatest part of Ed's
career was yet to come since he not only would have continued to pursue new
research goals, but perhaps more importantly Ed would have been a senior
member of the neurobiology research community who could have provided
direction and perspective to his past associates and to those who would
have continued to flock to the Laboratory of Neurophysiology to learn all
that was offered there. We will all miss Edward Vaughn Evarts.

Jerome N. Sanes
Section on Human Motor Control
Medical Neurology Branch
National Institute of Neurological
and Communicative Disorders and Stroke
Bethesda, Maryland

SECTION I
MOTOR UNIT ACTIVITY

THE PATTERN-RELATED MODIFICATIONS OF CONTRACTILE

RESPONSE OF HUMAN SKELETAL MUSCLE

V. S. Gurfinkel and Yu. S. Levik

Institute for Problems of Information Transmission
Ac. Sci. of the USSR
Moscow, USSR

The motor system of vertebrates produces the great variety of movements, but all forms of motor activity are based predominantly on two types of muscular contraction: the sustained maintenance of low tension (postural or tonic mode) and short bursts of activity (phasic mode). The problem of interrelation between two types of activity was discussed in physiology for many years. In this paper we want to discuss not the differences on the level of regulatory mechanisms but only on the level of muscles as actuators. It is known that some invertebrates have separate tonic and phasic muscles, which differ by innervation, structure of myofibrils, contractile proteins etc. Lower vertebrates more often have not tonic muscles but only tonic fibres in mixed muscles. Mammalian muscles consist of phasic (twitch) fibers only, but these fibers are heterogeneous (fast and slow).

It is often assumed that slow-twitch mammalian fibers are analogous to the tonic fibers of lower vertebrate, so posture maintenance and movements execution are performed by different motor units (MU). But differences in the MUs properties can be of limited use only. The existence of fixed recruitment order restricts the possibility of the independent activation of MUs with necessary properties. This control problem can be solved by additional mechanism capable to modify the contractile properties of already active fibers.

This paper is devoted to our research of the modifications of the contractile properties of human muscles during simulation of tonic and phasic modes of muscular work. These modifications of muscle properties were studied both in electrically evoked and voluntary contractions.

Experiments were performed in the m. flexor digitorum sublimis of the right arm. The motor point producing more or less isolated contraction of muscle portion flexing the ring finger was stimulated by superficial 5 x 5 mm electrode, the second electrode was fixed at the wrist. Rectangular pulses (1 ms, 30-60 V) were used. During electrical stimulation the muscle developed force and the second phalanx of the finger pressed on metal ring. This pressure was transferred on rigid (cross section 7 x 7 mm) steel measuring beam with semi-conductive strain guages. In other set of experiments the contractile properties of the muscle were also determined by measuring responses to the electrical stimulation, but these responses were preceded by voluntary contraction, the strength and duration of which were prescribed by an instruction.

The frequency of MUs during posture maintenance is known to be rather low, therefore their muscle fibers do not develop a fused contraction but produce an unfused one. It was also shown that in posture maintenance the same MUs are active over long time periods without "rotation". Accordingly, to stimulate the postural type of activity we have used the electrical stimulation of 10 pps and train durations of 1.0-1.5 m. The results of the study of such sustained unfused tetanus were published elsewhere (Gurfinkel and Levik, 1979, 1984). It was shown that in the sustained unfused tetanus three phases with significant differences can by distinguished: the initial plateau (phase I), the period of increased oscillations of force (phase II) and the period of slow increase of the mean force along with the simultaneous significant decrease of force oscillations (phase III). Let us discuss muscle properties during the phase III in more detail. In addition to 2-5-fold decrease of the force oscillations for this phase is typical a significant increase of half-relaxation time $T_{0.5}$ (up to 30-50 ms with respect to $T_{0.5}$ in phase II); a "shoulder" or "angle" appears on the relaxation curve. Muscle reacts on an additional pulse in the input train by so-called "catch-like" phenomenon. These changes point to the essential rearrangements in functioning of the contractile machinery. We supposed that in phase III the muscle works more efficiently. This was tested by direct measurements of the intramuscular temperature during isometric tension maintenance (Gurfinkel and Levik, 1981). 90 s muscle work under blood arrest conditions increases the intramuscular temperature by 0.5-0.7°C. The specific rate of heat production at the beginning of tetanus was equal to 60-70 mW/g, during the phase II it rose up to 120 mW/g and to the 40th-90th s (phase III) decreased to 30-40 mW/g. It has to be stressed that fall of heat production was not accompanied by a decrease of tension; as a rule the level of force was constant or increasing. As a result, the isometric economy of contraction increased 2-6-fold. It is interesting to note that these differences in economy between "fresh" muscle and a muscle in phase III are of the same order as the differences between the fast and slow mammalian muscles. So, during prolonged muscle activity (but before fatigue is developed) its properties shift toward those of slow muscles, therefore it can be assumed that muscle properties during phase III are well adjusted to the postural mode of activity.

These data were obtained under electrical stimulation. It was not clear if similar modifications take place during the natural asynchronous tonic activity. So we tried to checkout our data in the conditions of voluntary muscle contraction. The subject was asked to maintain a constant force (25-30% MVC) for 1-1.5 m using the visual feedback from the oscilloscope. On the end of voluntary contraction the electrical stimulation of about 10 pps was superimposed; the subject was instructed to relax with the beginning of stimulation. The stimulation lasted 1-2 s. The characteristics of electrically evoked contractions after preceding voluntary tonic activity were the same as after prolonged electrically evoked unfused tetanus (Figure 1). The changes of contractile properties of muscle under prolonged natural or artificial activation seem to be functionally significant. In fact, for postural mode of activity it is desirable to have a muscle with high resistance to fatigue, high economy, large stiffness in active state, insensitivity to small frequency variations. For this type of activity the velocity of tension development, the shortening velocity and power output are not so essential.

These changes in contractile properties of muscle arise under two conditions: the activation of muscle must be prolonged and continuous while the activating frequency must be relatively low. If the patterns of activation differ from those typical for postural mode, some other modifications arise. Under the activation simulating the phasic activity these changes are the same as in first 10-20 s of unfused tetanus. The contractile properties remain more similar to these of fast fibers: the twitch

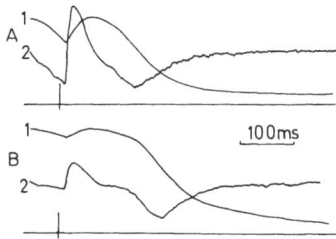

Fig. 1. Relaxation in isometric unfused tetanus evoked after voluntary
contraction. (A) after 10 s of voluntary contraction; (B) after
60 s. Stimulation frequency 10 pps. (1) isometric force; (2)
time derivative of force; (lower trace) stimulation mark of the
last pulse in train.

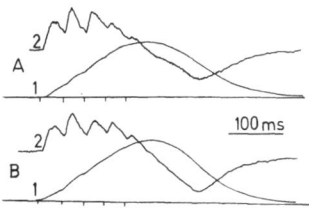

Fig. 2. Mechanical response of muscle on the 1st and 120th trains of
stimuli; interpulse intervals in trains 40 ms, frequency of trains
0.5 s^{-1}. (A) response on the 1st train; (B) response on the 120th
train. (1) isometric force; (2) time derivative of force; (lower
trace) stimulation marks.

force, relaxation rate and shortening velocity increase and remain increased (Figure 2). The muscle in this state has high work-producing
ability, i.e., the capability to fast splitting of ATP, and the ability for
follow the changes of input frequency (absence of prominent hysteresis
properties).

So we suggest that skeletal muscles can work efficiently both in
postural and phasic modes not only because of the existence of slow and
fast MUs, but also because of the ability of the muscle to modify it contractile properties depending on the duration of activity and the distribution of interpulse intervals. Such "operative" control of muscle properties can be based on the calcium-dependent phosphorilation of some muscle
proteins, in particular, myosin light chains (LC_2) (Kushmerick and Crow,
1983; Moor and Stull, 1984).

REFERENCES

Gurfinkel, V. S., and Levik, Yu. S., 1979, The successive phases of the
        sustained unfused tetanus of human skeletal muscle, Biofizika,
        23:758 (in Russian).
Gurfinkel, V. S., and Levik, Yu. S., 1984, The force of isometric twitch in
        different phases of unfused tetanus, Biofizika, 29:139 (in Russian).
Gurfinkel, V. S., and Levik, Yu. S., 1981, The economy of the muscle con-
        traction during the unfused tetanus," Biofizika, 26:371 (in
        Russian).

Kushmerick, M. J., Crow, M. T., 1983, Regulation of energetics and mechanics by myosin light chain phosphorylation in fast-twitch skeletal muscle, Federation Proc., 42:14.

Moor, R. L., and Stull, J. T., 1984, Myosin light chain phosphorylation in fast and slow skeletal muscle in situ., Am.J.Physiol., 277:C462.

MOTOR UNIT DISCHARGES IN INTEROSSEUS DORSALIS

PRIMUS MUSCLE DURING VOLUNTARY MOVEMENTS

D. Kosarov, A. Gydikov, and A. Kossev

Central Laboratory of Biophysics
Bulgarian Academy of Sciences
Sofia, Bulgaria

Studies of the firing pattern of the motor units (MUs) upon different voluntary movements are restricted by the inadequacy of the current methods. Summing up of the impulses of different MUs in higher muscle efforts disturbs the separation of the trains from single units. To overcome this obstacle selective electrodes were used. However, the more selective is an electrode, the more susceptible it is to changes in the parameters of the selected impulses when changing its position in respect to the MU. Thus the study of the MU-impulses upon greater angle of movement, when the leading-off electrodes are displaced from their initial position is difficult.

METHODS

The experiments were performed with five healthy subjects aged between 35 and 57 years, without deviations in the standard electromyogram (EMG). The firing pattern of twelve MUs was investigated, comprising the MUs of interossei dorsales dig. I muscles of both hands. The selective cutaneous EMG was led-off by concentric (Gydikov et al., 1981) and linear branched electrodes (Gydikov et al., 1984) (Figure 1). An elastic plate suitable to be caught by the proximal phalanxes of the thumb and index fingers was supplied with a strain gauge. The tensogram was parallelly led-off by the same "Medelec" equipment as the EMG. When executing the movement the thumb was fixed on a straight line coming from the forearm, the basis of the proximal phalanx of the index finger pressing the elastic plate. According to the instruction the subject varied the velocity of the movement comprising 30° rotation. Thus the maximal possible muscle tension against the elastic resistance was reached. The latter was measured in N. The inter-impulse intervals were measured in ms and the instant frequency was calculated. In many cases two MUs in one trial were registered.

RESULTS

Depending on the time parameter of the increasing muscle tension (0.15-4.00 s) the MUs of the muscle investigated showed the following type of behavior:

A   **B**

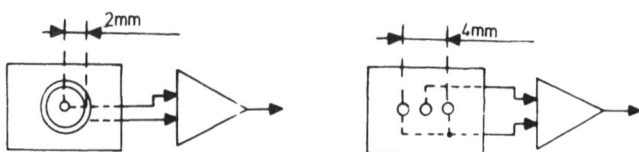

Fig. 1.   Selective surface electrodes.

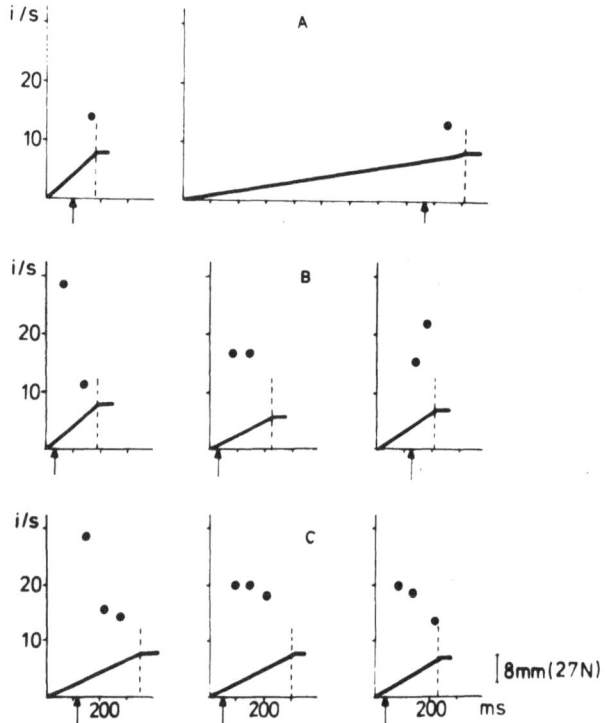

Fig. 2.   Frequencygram of a selected MU and mechanogram of the movement
          against elastic resistance during quick movements. (A) firing of
          the MU by two impulses. (B) firing of the MU by three impulses.
          (C) firing of the MU by four impulses.

1. The MU fired only one impulse during the rising of the tension. It
   happened most frequently in the cases of high-threshold MUs, which had
   not time to fire again during the quick rise of the tension and before
   its stabilization at a high level.
2. The MU fired twice (Figure 2-A). They were both low-threshold MUs at
   very short rise of the tension and high-threshold MUs at shorter movements and shorter interimpulse interval (I-I). It is characteristic
   of the MUs of m. interosseus dors. I that the instant frequency was
   lower in average than the corresponding one for the MUs of m. biceps
   brachii (Gydikov et al., 1985).
3. The MU fired three times. This is marked by two I-I which match or
   differ (Figure 2-B). In short term of increase of the tension two of
   the possibilities occur in equal proportions: First I-I -short, second
   I-I long or two equal I-Is. The third possibility (first I-I longer
   than the second I-I) was rarely observed.

4. The MU succeeded to fire four times (Figure 2-C). This was found upon movements lasting 0.4-1.0 s. The variety of the possible consequences rose, but beginning with first I-I - long, second I-I - short, and equality of both intervals was frequently observed.
5. The MU fired with more impulses (Figure 3). This was established upon movements longer than 1.0 s (the self pacing of all the subjects never exceeded 4.0 s). In most cases the chain of impulses started with the longest interval in the chain. After it the instant frequency tended to increase, reaching a steady level before or at the end of the movement. In many cases a short I-I came after the middle of the movement to disturb the evenness of the picture. Very often all the firing exhibited a similar mean frequency from the beginning to the end. However, it was not so difficult to find that the middle part of the movement was completed with lower dispersion of the length of the I-Is than the beginning and the end (Figure 4).

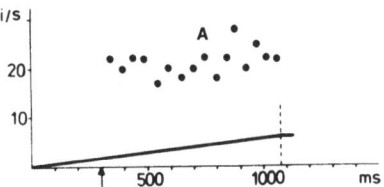

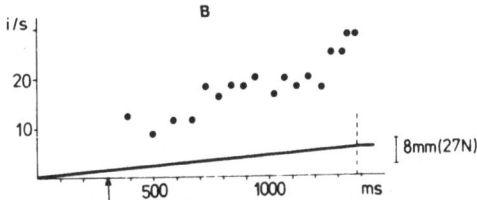

Fig. 3. Frequencygram of a selected MU during long-lasting movements, and the mechanogram of the movement against elastic resistance. (A) firing of the MU with constant mean frequency. (B) firing of the MU with an increasing frequency.

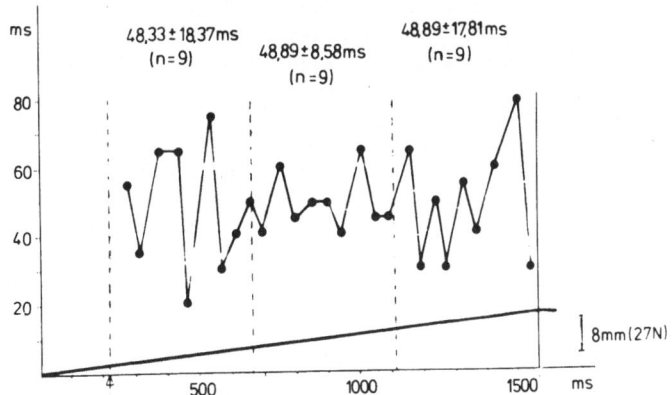

Fig. 4. An example of the firing of a selected MU with a constant mean frequency of firing during all the movement against elastic resistance, but with different dispersion of the I-Is in the beginning, the middle and the end of the movement.

DISCUSSION

The rise of the muscle force in voluntary contraction is due to several factors. The first one is the recruitment of more and more MUs. This results from the difference in the thresholds of firing of the alpha-motoneurons in the motor nucleus of the muscle. The ranging of the thresholds follows the size of the alpha-motoneurons (after Henneman, 1957, and later) and the type of the motor task (Burke, 1981, and others). The order of recruitment is therefore relatively fixed, and may be changed. This change might occur also between neurons not so similar in size, and it is determined statistically (Gydikov and Kosarov, 1972a). The alpha-motoneuron threshold in man is measured indirectly by the level of the muscle tension at the very beginning of the MU-firing. With the increase of the speed of the rising force the threshold decreases (Gydikov and Kosarov, 1972b; Freund et al., 1975; Büdingen and Freund, 1976; Kosarov et al., 1978; Gydikov et al., 1985). At the fastest possible muscle contraction, in the so called ballistic movements, the recruitment of all MUs may (and must) occur at zero tension measured (Desmdt and Godaux, 1977a).

The second factor for the increase in the muscle force at voluntary contractions is the rise of the MU-impulse frequency. At constant isometric tension this frequency is almost constant too. At higher tension the frequency is also higher. At continuously increasing tension, without steps, the frequency is usually higher (Tokizane and Shimazu, 1964; Gydikov and Kosarov, 1974; Freund et al., 1975; Monster and Chan, 1977). Under some restrictions, however (i.e., in quick, ballistic movements - Desmedt and Godaux, 1977a, 1978) the frequency of firing decreased during the movement.

The third factor is the real pattern of the MU-firing, i.e., the duration of the consecutive I-Is. Gurfinkel and Levik (1973) showed the complex dependence of the mechanical output on the superposition of the successive contractions of the MU. Therefore not only the mean frequency of firing, but also the instant frequency are of importance. This holds true particularly for the short, speedy movements (Desmedt and Godaux, 1977a,b, 1978). This factor plays a basic role in the transient processes of the MUs, switching them on and off (Gurfinkel et al., 1970; Gurfinkel et al., 1972, 1977; Gydikov and Kosarov, 1972b).

In the present paper the ability of the MUs of m. interosseus dors I to fire according to the velocity of the movement was proved, as Gydikov et al. (1985) had made for the MUs of the biceps brachii muscle. There are however some quantitative differences. At fastest movements these differences are minimal. It means that the movements executed in time-deficit conditions are similar in programing never mind which muscle is activated - distal or proximal. In long-lasting movements the differences are more distinct. It proved that the MUs of the distal muscle did not show a marked transient process upon switching on - the first I-I might be the longest one in the series. We may consider the biomechanics responsible for this difference. Biceps brachii muscle has to move a peripheral link with a significant inertness. The interosseus muscle has to move only a finger. It appeared that the beginning of the contraction of its MUs did not need any potentiation of their biomechanical effect using short initial I-Is.

In case of some MUs of m. interosseus dors. I the dynamic addition to the frequency of firing brought to the appearance of a plateau-frequency. As quicker was the movement, as earlier was the stabilization of the plateau-frequency. These results confirm the results of our previous paper (Kosarov et al., 1976) on the existence of two types of MUs in m. inter-

10

osseus dors. I according to their peculiarities in frequency/tension relationships in isometric conditions.

REFERENCES

Büdingen, H. J., and Freund, J. 1976, The relationship between the rate of rise of isometric tension and motor unit recruitment in a human forearm muscle, Pflüggers Arch., 362:61-67.

Burke, R. E., 1981, Motor unit recruitment: What are the critical factors? in: "Motor Unit Types, Recruitment and Plasticity in Health and Disease," J. E. Desmedt (ed.), Karger, Basel.

Desmedt, J. E., and Godaux, E., 1977a, Ballistic contractions in man: characteristic recruitment pattern of single motor units of the tibialis anterior muscle, J.Physiol.(Lond.), 264:673-693.

Desmedt, J. E., and Godaux, E., 1977b, Fast motor units are not preferentially activated in rapid voluntary contractions in man, Nature (Lond.), 267:717-719.

Desmedt, J. E., and Godaux, E., 1978, Ballistic contractions in fast and slow human muscles: discharge patterns of single motor units, J.Physiol.(Lond.), 285:185-196.

Freund, J., and Büdingen, H. J., 1975, Motor unit activity during voluntary contractions of human forearm muscles, Expl.Brain Res., 23, Suppl., p.72.

Gurfinkel, V. S., and Levik, Y.S., 1973, Dependence of the muscle contraction on the consequence of the activating impulses, Biofizika, 18:116-131 (in Russian).

Gurfinkel, V. S., Mirskyi, M. L., Tarko, A. M., and Surguladze, T. D., 1972, Work of the motor units upon the initiation of the muscle tension, Biofizika, 17:303-309 (in Russian).

Gurfinkel, V. S., Surguladze, T. D., Mirskyi, M. L., and Tarko, A. M., 1970, Work of the human motor units in rhythmic movements, Biofizika, 15:1090-1095 (in Russian).

Gydikov, A., and Kosarov, D., 1972a, Volume conduction of the potentials from separate motor units in human muscle, Electromyography, 12:127-147.

Gydikov, A., and Kosarov, D., 1927b, Extraterritorial potential field of impulses from separate motor units in human muscles, Electromyography, 12:283-305.

Gydikov, A., and Kosarov, D., 1974, Some features of different motor units in human biceps brachii, Pflüggers Arch., 374:75-88.

Gydikov, A., Kossev, A., Kosarov, D., and Kostov, K., 1985, Investigation of single motor units firing during movements against elastic resistance, p.68, in: "Abstracts of the 5th International Symposium on Motor Control, Varna, 10-15.06. 1985".

Gydikov, A., Kossev, A., Trayanova, N., and Radicheva, N., 1985, Selective recording of single motor unit potentials, EMG Clin.Neurophysiol. (in press).

Gydikov, A., Kostov, K., and Gatev, P., Mechanical properties and discharge frequencies of single motor units in human m. biceps brachii, in: "Neural and Mechanical Control of Movement," M. Kumamoto (ed.), Yamagushi Shoten, Kyoto.

Henneman, E., 1957, Relation between size of neurones and their susceptibility to discharge, Science, 126:1345-1346.

Kosarov, D., Rokotova, N. A. Shapkov, Y. T., and Anissimova, N. P. 1978, Activity of single motor units in voluntary control of isometric muscle tension on man, Acta Physiol.Pharmacol.Bulg., 4:3-11.

Monster, A. W., and Chan, H., 1977, Isometric force production by motor units of extensor digitorum communis muscle in man, J.Neurophysiol., 40:1432-1443.

Tokizane, T., and Shimazu, H. 1964, Functional differentiation of human skeletal muscle, in: "Corticalization and Spinalization of Movement," Ch. C. Thomas, Springfield, Ill.

THE USE OF LOW AND HIGH THRESHOLD UNITS DURING

VOLUNTARY CONTRACTION AND LOCOMOTION

L. Grimby

Department of Neurology
Karolinska Hospital
Stockholm, Sweden

The aim of the studies was to determine how single motor units of different types are used during activities of daily living in man. The extensor digitorum brevis muscle (EDB) was selected for study for technical reasons. The EDB muscle consists of about 50% type I and 50% type II fibers. For details see Grimby and Hannerz 1977; Borg, Grimby and Hannerz 1978; Grimby, Hannerz and Hedman 1981, Grimby 1984.

METHODS

Recordings of just one muscle fiber could not be used for studies of single motor units during movements because of electrode displacement. Instead multifiber recordings were used in muscles in which the number of units was decreased or the muscle fiber density within the units increased:

1. In the EDB muscle there were clusters of muscle fibers innervated by one and the same motoneurone. When a recording electrode, made up from two 20-100 μ wires, was inserted into such a cluster and retained by means of a hook, recordings of just this motor unit could be achieved also during natural movements. Clusters of sufficient size were scarce in ordinary subjects and usually only a few motor units could be studied in each subject. In three members of the research group, however, a large number of units could be studied. The three subjects had taken part in several electromyographic studies which presumably had caused repeated lesions to the terminal nerve twigs and muscle fibers and consequent collateral sprouting and increased muscle fiber density within the units.
2. In certain normal subjects there was an accessory innervation of just a few EDB units. These units could easily be studied during lidocain blockade of the main innervation.

There might be sources of error in the two techniques used; lesions to the periphery of a motoneurone might change its firing properties; blocking of the EDB innervation reduces the proprioceptive afferent activity that is known to play a part for the motoneurone firing. However, the findings were reproduced with both techniques and should be conclusive since the sources of error were different.

AXONAL CONDUCTION VELOCITY

The type of the motor unit was identified by its axonal conduction
velocity. The conduction velocity of the axon was calculated as illustrated in Figure 1 A–C. The axonal conduction velocity was determined for
144 units. The conduction velocities ranged from 30 ms to 58 ms as shown
in the histograms in Figure 1 D and E. About half of the units had conduction velocities between 40 and 45 m/s and there seemed to be a unimodal
distribution. There was no significant difference between the histogram of
clustered units (Figure 1 D) and that of accessory units (Figure 1 E).

SUSTAINED VOLUNTARY TENSION

All 144 units were studied during isometric voluntary contraction
slowly increasing from zero to maximal tension. Each motor unit had its
particular recruitment tension and its particular minimum rate for tonic
firing. The units with the lowest thresholds were recruited already before
any tension was recorded and could fire tonically at rates as low as
7–8 Hz. These units could be driven voluntarily at 10–20 Hz for apparently
unlimited periods of time. The units with the highest thresholds were
recruited at about 80% of the maximal tension and fired tonically only at
rates above 20 Hz as illustrated in Figure 2. Extraordinary effort was
required to maintain such high tensions. Tonic firing of high threshold
units must be very rare.

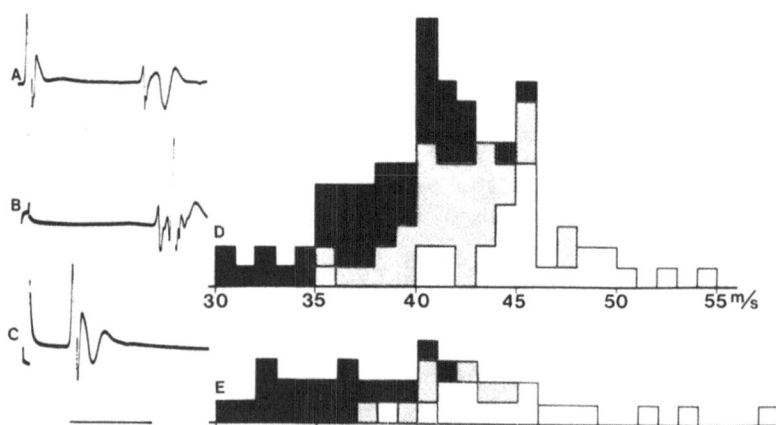

Fig. 1. Left column shows calculation of axonal conduction velocity. The
         potentials of two units could be identified during maximal volun-
         tary contraction (A) and after supramaximal proximal electrical
         nerve stimulation (B). One of them could be identified also after
         distal nerve stimulation (C). The conduction velocity was calcul-
         ated from the latency difference between proximal and distal
         stimulation and the distance between the stimulation points. The
         motor unit with the large amplitude potential had a conduction
         velocity of 35 m/s. The unit with the small amplitude potential
         seemed to conduct more rapidly but its conduction velocity could
         not be exactly determined. Time bar 10 ms. Right column shows
         the relation between conduction velocity and threshold for clus-
         tered units (D) and accessory units (E). Filled squares denote
         low threshold units (that could be driven for apparently unlimited
         periods of time). Open squares high threshold units responding
         mainly phasically, dotted squares denote intermediates.

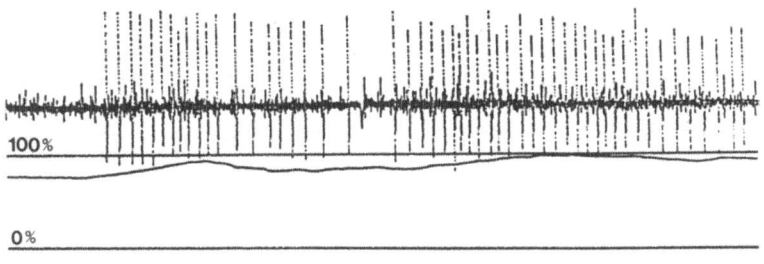

Fig. 2. The firing of a high threshold unit during sustained isometric
voluntary contraction. Upper trace EMG. Lower trace tension.
Straight lines denote zero and maximal tension (defined as the toe
dorsiflexor tension evoked by supramaximal tetanization of the
peroneal nerve). The test unit had a threshold tension about 80%
and a minimal rate higher than 20 Hz. Time bar 1 s.

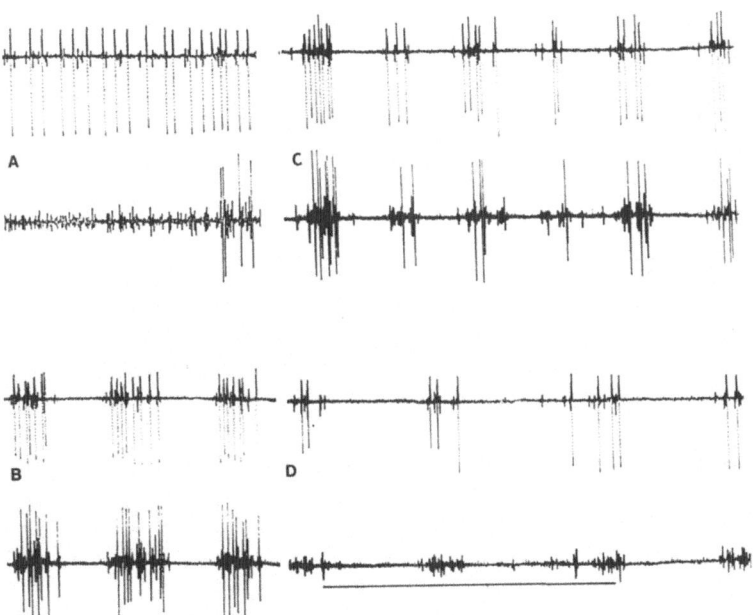

Fig. 3. The change in relative roles of low and high threshold units on
change in mode of voluntary contraction. One low threshold unit
(upper trace in A-D) and one high threshold unit (lower trace in
A-D) were recorded simultaneously. During slowly increasing
isometric tension (A) the low threshold units fired selectively
until it was close to its maximal rate that was 30 Hz. During
vigorous toe waving (B) both units responded in high frequency
bursts. When the subject was told to wave the toes at maximal
rate but minimal amplitude (C) the number of discharges per cycle
decreased in a similar way in both units. Selective activation of
one of the units occurred but very occasionally. Only when the
rate of toe waving was decreased (D) the low threshold unit could
be used selectively as during sustained tension. Time bar 1 s.

The histograms in Figure 1 show that there was a correlation between
threshold and axonal conduction velocity as implied by the "size principle". Units with such low thresholds that they could be driven tonically
for apparently unlimited periods of time had conduction velocities between
30 and 45 m/s. Motor units with such high thresholds that they mainly
responded phasically had conduction velocities between 40 and 58 m/s.
Intermediate threshold units had, however, overlapping conduction velocities.

VOLUNTARY MOVEMENTS

The changes in firing on changes from sustained voluntary tension to
rapid voluntary movement were studied in 40 units. The differences in
firing between the motor unit types decreased with the rapidity of the
movement as shown in Figure 3. During toe waving at 3-4 Hz, that was the
maximal rate that could be maintained by most subjects, all units fired in
very similar ways. High threshold units responded as readily as low threshold units. Selective activation of one motor unit type did not occur
systematically. Power was regulated by the number of discharges rather
than by recruitment.

LOCOMOTION

Long-term recordings showed that the EDB-muscle was active mainly
during locomotion. Recruitment and firing rates increased with increasing
speed of locomotion. When asked to walk at free speed most subjects chose

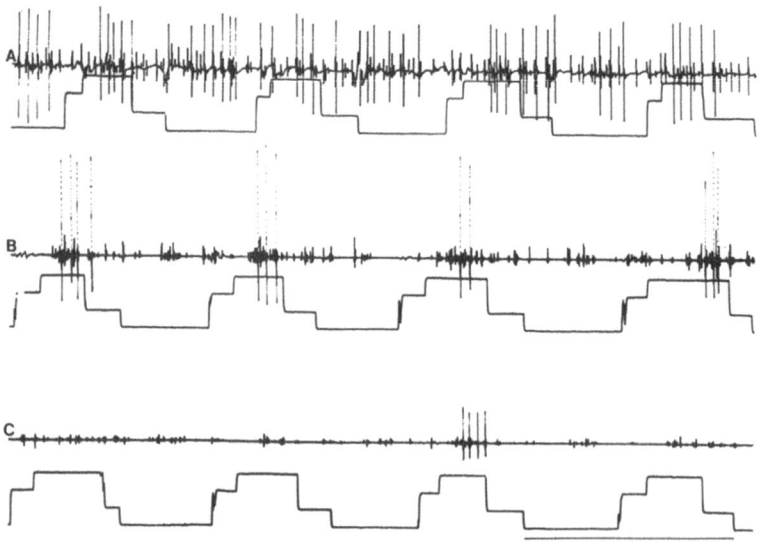

Fig. 4. The use of one low threshold unit (A) one intermediate unit (B)
and one high threshold units (C) during walking 55-60 c/min.
Upper traces in A,B,C EMG. Lower traces signals from foot-
switches; high amplitude upward deflexion denotes pressure on the
whole sole; intermediate amplitude denotes pressure only on the
heel; low amplitude denotes pressure only on the anterior part of
the sole. The low threshold unit fired tonically, the intermediate unit phasically in each step cycle and the high threshold
unit only in a diverging stride. Time bar 1 s.

50-60 cycles per minute. The use of a motor unit during that speed of walking should reflect its long term use better than any other single test. Single motor units were studied during free walking in 40 experiments. The recording electrodes were connected to the main amplifier either wireless of by means of a cable permitting 40 m locomotion.

Low threshold units fired 5-10 times in each step cycle at intervals between 100-40 ms corresponding to firing rates between 10 and 25 Hz, (Figure 4A). Intermediate motor units fired in most step cycles but only a few times per cycle at intervals between 70 and 40 ms corresponding to firing rates between 15 and 25 Hz (Figure B). High threshold units did not participate in the ordinary step cycle, but fired when the speed of walking was increased, direction of walking was changed or obstacles were avoided, etc., i.e., during corrective movements. Usually the number of discharges in each burst was only 1-4 and the intervals between discharges as short as 30 and 100 Hz (Figure C).

REFERENCES

Grimby, L., and Hannerz, J. 1977, Firing rate and recruitment order of toe extensor motor units in different modes of voluntary contraction, J.Physiol., 264:865.
Borg, J., Grimby, L. and Hannerz, J. 1978, Axonal conduction velocity and voluntary discharge properties of individual short toe extensor motor in man, J.Physiol., 277:143.
Grimby, L., Hannerz, J., and Hedman, B. 1981, The fatigue and voluntary discharge properties of single motor units in man, J.Physiol., 316:545.
Grimby, L., 1984, Firing properties of single human motor units during locomotion, J.Physiol., 346:195.

MEASUREMENT AND CHARACTERISTICS OF RECURRENT IPSPs

PRODUCED BY STIMULATION OF SINGLE MOTOR AXONS

T. M. Hamm*, C. -S. Yuan, S. -I. Sasaki, and D. G. Stuart

Department of Physiology, University of Arizona
Health Sciences Center
Tucson, Arizona, U.S.A.

The study of the properties and organization of spinal synaptic pathways has benefited greatly from the use of techniques for recording the postsynaptic potentials produced by activity of single neurons, such as the method of spike-triggered averaging (see Kirkwood and Sears, 1980). We have combined spike-triggered averaging with methods for stimulating single motor axons in order to study the recurrent pathway to spinal motoneurons, a pathway which has generated considerable interest in its organization and functional significance since the pioneering studies of Renshaw (1941, 1946; for review, see Baldissera et al., 1981). In this report, these methods will be described and the characteristics of homonymous recurrent inhibitory postsynaptic potentials (RIPSPs) evoked by stimulation of single motor axons innervating the medial gastrocnemius (MG) muscle of the cat will be presented.

Two methods have been employed to stimulate single motor axons. The first was adapted from the method of Zealear and Crandall (1982; see also Yuan et al., 1983). In this technique, a stepping motor is used to advance a glass micropipette filled with 2 M potassium citrate into the MG fascicle of the sciatic nerve. For this purpose, a short length of the sciatic (approx. 2 cm) is stabilized by being pinned to a layer of wax on a stable platform. Penetrations of axons in their myelin sheaths are indicated by positive-going antidromic action potentials in response to stimulation of the MG nerve (cf. Tasaki, 1952; Zealear and Crandall, 1982). Once an axon is impaled, it is identified as a motor axon by recording an action potential extracellularly in the ventral roots and a muscle-unit twitch in response to stimulating the axon, using 0.1-0.5 ms pulses of anodal current.

The second method is modified from that of Taylor and Stephens (1976; see also Stalberg and Trontelj, 1979). A fine bipolar EMG electrode is used to stimulate motor axons in nerve branches within the MG muscle. The electrode is advanced manually in steps through the muscle tissue. At each site, 0.1 ms stimulus pulses are applied to the electrode and the ability to stimulate a single motor axon (usually by activation of one or more of

*Present Address: Barrow Neurological Institute, Division of Neurobiology, St. Joseph's Hospital and Medical Center, 350 W. Thomas Road, Phoenix, Arizona 85013, U.S.A.

its collaterals) is judged by extracellular ventral root recordings. These recordings are obtained from three ventral root segments (the rostral and caudal parts of L7 and S1) placed on monopolar electrodes. With this recording configuration, the potentials of single motor axons can be distinguished in single traces. Consequently, the unitary nature of recorded spikes can be judged by their all-or-one character at stimulus threshold. If a single axon can be stimulated at strengths of 2.5-3 times threshold without activating other axons, then that axon is selected for study.

Both of these techniques have been used with averaging methods to record single-axon RIPSPs. Two types of preparations have been used. In the first, the cat is anesthetized with a mixture of chloralose and urethane. In the second, the animal is allowed to become unanesthetized following ischemic brain destruction by occlusion of the carotid and vertebral arteries under anesthesia with halothane and a mixture of oxygen and nitrous oxide. In both preparations, the dorsal roots (L6-S2) are sectioned. MG motoneurons are impaled with glass micropipettes filled with 2M potassium citrate. Following penetration, single-axon RIPSPs are evoked by stimulating the test motor axon at rates of 6-7 Hz and the ensuing potentials are collected using a signal averager.

Examples of single-axon RIPSPs are shown in Figure 1. Most notable are the long time courses of these potentials, which have a duration comparable to that of composite RIPSPs. Eccles et al.(1954) suggested that the long duration of RIPSPs might be due to the repetitive discharge of Renshaw cells which occurs in response to an antidromic volley. While short bursts of spikes by Renshaw cells may occur in response to activation of single motoneurons (Ross et al., 1975, 1976; Van Keulen, 1981), such bursts are not as intense and longlasting as in the case of bursts evoked by composite volleys. Consequently, our findings suggest that the long duration of RIPSPs may be due, in part, to the time course of the post-synaptic potentials produced in motoneurons by single impulses of Renshaw cells. This conclusion is in agreement with some of the recordings by Van Keulen (1981) of motoneuron IPSPs produced by the discharge of single Renshaw cells.

A feature of several of the single-axon RIPSPs which we have recorded is the presence of two "peaks" in the potential, suggestive of two components (Figure 1C and D). Cullheim and Kellerth (1981) have demonstrated two components of composite RIPSPs, a short-duration component which is sensitive to strychnine, presumably mediated by glycine, and a long-duration component which is sensitive to bicuculline and picrotoxin, presumably mediated by GABA. Whether the two apparent components of our single-axon RIPSPs represent the components seen by Cullheim and Kellerth, or are due to other factors, such as the pattern of Renshaw cell discharge, remains a topic for investigation in future studies.

Single-axon RIPSPs were found to be quite variable in amplitude, in part depending upon the use of anesthesia. As shown in Table 1, the amplitude of RIPSPs in unanesthetized ischemic-decapitate preparations was approximately three times as great as that of RIPSPs in cats anesthetized with chloralose-urethane. This finding is in agreement with the studies of Haase and Van der Meulen (1961) and Biscoe and Krnjevic (1963) on the effects of chloralose on the recurrent inhibitory pathway. Apart from the differences in amplitude, the characteristics of the RIPSPs in the two preparations were quite similar. The long duration of the RIPSPs which was noted in Figure 1 is evident in the range and mean value of half-widths in Table 1.

The present report (see also Yuan et al., 1985) demonstrates the feasibility of recording single-axon RIPSPs and suggests their potential in

Table 1. Characteristics of Single-Axon RIPSPs

Preparation	Amplitude* (μV)	Latency (ms)	Rise-time (ms)	Half-width (ms)
Chloralose-urethane	12.0 ± 6.7 (3.1-27.7)	3.0 ± 2.2 (1.0-7.3)	5.9 ± 3.3 (1.0-9.9)	24.1 ± 12.4 (8.6-41.8)
Ischemic decapitate	35.3 ± 28.0 (13.3-134.3)	3.2 ± 2.1 (0.7-9.2)	5.7 ± 2.4 (3.6-10.5)	23.1 ± 14.7 (7.6-51.2)

*Values are presented as mean ± standard deviation with range of values in parentheses.

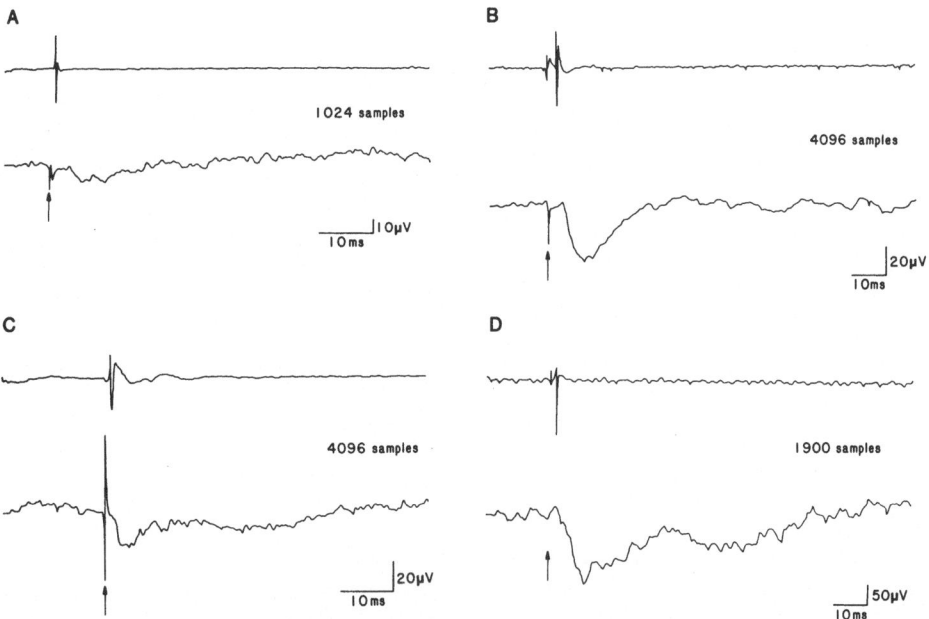

Fig. 1. Recordings of single-axon RIPSPs. In this figure, the top trace of each set is an averaged extracellular recording from a ventral root segment and the lower trace is an averaged intracellular recording from an MG motoneuron. The arrow below each set shows the time at which the stimulus was applied which evoked the spike in the ventral-root recording the the RIPSP. (A) and (C) are from chloralose-urethane preparations, and (B) and (D) are from ischemic decapitate preparations. A trace of EMG is evident following the ventral-root spike in (C).

the study of the organization of recurrent pathways from motoneurons. Elsewhere, we have reported preliminary results which indicate that the incidence of single-axon RIPSPs within the MG motor nucleus is dependent upon the proximity of the two motoneurons involved in the test (Sasaki et al., 1985). It is our expectation that future studies with the presently described techniques will provide important information concerning the properties and organization of recurrent inhibiton.

Acknowledgments

This work was supported by U.S.P.H.S. grants NS 07888 (to D.G.S.), NS/AM 17887 (to T.M.H.) and HL 07249 (To the Department of Physiology) and by travel awards from the U.S. and Bulgarian Academies of Sciences (to T.M.H. and D.G.S.). We would like to thank Dr S. Vanden Noven and Professor U. Windhorst for their assistance.

REFERENCES

Baldissera, F., Hultborn, H., and Illert, M., 1981, Integration in spinal neuronal systems, in: "Handbook of Physiology, Sec. 1, Vol. II, The Nervous System: Motor Control, Part 1," V. B. Brooks, ed., Am. Physiol. Soc., Bethesda.

Biscoe, J. T. and Krnjevic, K., 1963, Chloralose and the activity of Renshaw cells, Exp.Neurol., 6:395.

Cullheim, S. and Kellerth, J. -O, 1981, Two kinds of recurrent inhibition of cat spinal α-motoneurones as differentiated pharmacologically, J.Physiol.(Lond.), 312:209.

Eccles, J. C., Fatt, P., and Koketsu, K., 1954, Cholinergic and inhibitory synapses in a pathway from motor-axon collaterals to motoneurons, J.Physiol.(Lond.), 126:524.

Haase, J. and Van der Meulen, J. P., 1961, Die spezifische Wirkung der Chloralose auf die recurrente Inhibition tonisches Motoneurone, Pflug.Archiv., 274:272.

Kirkwood, P. A. and Sears, T. A., 1980, The measurement of synaptic connections in the mammalian nervous system by means of spike-triggered averaging, in: "Spinal and Supraspinal Mechanisms of Voluntary Motor Control and Locomotion. Progr. in Clin. Neurophysiol., Vol. 8," J. Desmedt, ed., Karger, Basel.

Renshaw, B., 1941, Influence of discharge of motoneurons upon excitation of neighboring motoneurons, J.Neurophysiol., 4:167.

Renshaw, B., 1946, Central effects of centripetal impulses in axons of spinal ventral roots, J.Neurophysiol., 9:191.

Ross, H. G., Cleveland, S., and Haase, J., 1975, Contribution of single motoneurons to Renshaw cell activity, Neurosci.Lett., 1:105.

Ross, H. G., Cleveland, S., and Haase, J., 1976, Quantitative relation between discharge frequencies of a Renshaw cell and an intra-cellularly depolarized motoneuron, Neurosci.Lett., 3:129.

Sasaki, S. -I., Yuan, C. -S., Hamm, T. M., Windhorst, U., Vanden Noven, S., and Stuart, D. G., 1985, Topographic distribution of recurrent IPSPs to motoneurons supplying the medial gastrocnemius muscle of the cat, Soc.Neurosci.Abstr., 11:699.

Stalberg, E. and Trontelj, J., 1979, "Single Fibre Electromyography," Mirvalle, Woking.

Tasaki, I., 1952, Properties of myelinated fibers in frog sciatic nerve and in spinal cord as examined with microelectrodes, Jap.J.Physiol., 3:73.

Taylor, A. and Stephens, J. A., 1976, Study of human motor unit contractions by controlled intramuscular stimulation, Brain Res., 117:331.

Van Keulen, L., 1981, Autogenetic recurrent inhibition of individual spinal motoneurones of the cat, Neurosci.Lett., 21:197.

Yuan, C. -S., Hamm, T. M., Reinking, R. M., and Stuart, D. G., 1983, Selective activation of single type-identified muscle receptor axons, Soc.Neurosci.Abstr., 9:863.

Yuan, C. -S., Hamm, T. M., Sasaki, S., Windhorst, U., Vanden Noven, S., and Stuart, D. G., 1985, Characteristics of recurrent IPSPs produced by stimulation of single motor axons, Soc.Neurosci.Abstr., 11:699.

Zealear, D. L. and Crandall, W. F., 1982, Stimulating and recording from axons within their myelin sheaths: a stable and nondamaging method for studying single motor units, J.Neurosci.Meth., 5:47.

APPLICATION OF CROSS-SECTIONAL SINGLE-FIBER MICROCHEMISTRY

TO THE STUDY OF MOTOR-UNIT FATIGABILITY

P. M. Nemeth, T. M. Hamm*, D. A. Gordon
R. M. Reinking, and D. G. Stuart
Dept. of Neurology (P.M.N.), Washington University School
of Medicine, St. Louis, Missouri, and
Dept. of Physiology, University of Arizona Health Sciences
Center, Tucson, Arizona, U.S.A.

The glycogen-depletion technique for histologically identifying physiologically defined motor units, as proposed by Krnjevic and Miledi (1958) and first used by Edstrom and Kugelberg (1968), has provided a means of demonstrating associations between the physiological and biochemical properties of single motor units. Such associations have been demonstrated using largely qualitative histochemistry (e.g., Burke et al., 1971; Edstrom and Kugelberg, 1968; for review, Burke, 1981) but, most recently, quantitative biochemistry (Nemeth et al., 1981). The latter approach provides the advantage of yielding quantitative information on biochemical activites suitable for detailed comparison with physiological parameters. We have recently reported the development of a technique which permits biochemical analysis of cross-sections of fibers belonging to single mammalian motor units (Nemeth et al., 1985).

With the greater productivity afforded by this technique, it is now feasible to collect sufficient material to rigorously test for assocations between physiological and biochemical properties, within single motor units (viz., Nemeth et al., 1985) and both within and among groups of motor units of physiologically defined type. The present report provides preliminary results on relationships between fatigue resistance, as measured physiologically, and the activities of three enzymes (lactate dehydrogenase - LDH, a marker for anaerobic glycolysis, malate dehydrogenase - MDH, for the citric acid cycle and the malate-aspartate shuttle; and β hydroxyacyl CoA dehydrogenase-βOAC, for fatty-acid oxidation) in six physiologically identified fast-fatigable (FF) motor units from the tibialis posterior (TP) muscle of the cat.

The surgical procedures and physiological analyses were performed on anesthetized adult cats (halothane-nitrous oxide-oxygen followed by barbiturate). After a lumbosacral laminectomy and complete denervation of the left hindlimb, except for the TP muscle, motor axons were functionally isolated in ventral-root filaments and stimulated using 0.1 ms pulses. The activated motor units (1/muscle) were classified conventionally (Burke,

---

*Present address: Barrow Neurological Institute, Division of Neurobiology, St. Joseph's Hospital and Medical Center, 350 W. Thomas Road, Phoenix, Arizona 85013, U.S.A.

23

1981) according to twitch contraction time, profile of unfused tetanus ("sag" test) and force response during a 2 min fatigue test which consisted of 1/s 40 Hz stimulus trains of 330 ms duration. The fatigue test was continued for a total of 15 min for each FF unit to deplete it of its glycogen. Immediately thereafter, the muscle was removed and quickly frozen in liquid nitrogen (temperature reduced to approximately $-210°C$) and stored at $-70°C$ for subsequent analyses.

The biochemical and histochemical analyses were performed on transverse sections of muscle tissue, cut 16-18 μm thick on a cryostat. Alternate sections were processed for myosin ATPase (preincubation at pH 4.5), for the periodic acid-Schiff (PAS) reaction to identify glycogen-depleted fibers, and for analytical biochemistry. The latter sections were lyophilized for 24 hr (pressure less than 10^{-2} torr, temperature at $-38°C$).

Fibers of the depleted unit were identified using photographs of the PAS-stained sections as maps. The fibers for biochemistry were dissected under a stereomicroscope, from adjacent lyophilized unstained sections, weighed precisely on a quartz fiber torsion balance, and assayed for enzymes in microliter volumes of assay reagent, using the methods originally described by Lowry and Passaneau (1972). Multiple samples of each fiber were obtained from sequential lyophilized sections for the different assays.

Figure 1 shows the force and electromyographic (EMG) profiles of three FF units during the 2 min fatigue test. Part A of this Figure shows that one of the units displayed marked potentiation (greater than 130%) followed by a rapid decline in force. The two other units shown in A were more typical, showing little, if any, potentiation. The time course of the decline of force was quite different for these latter two units, despite the fact that the commonly used progressive fatigue index (force at 2 min divided by force at start of test) was similar for these and all other units studied (Table 1). For this reason, an alternative index of fatigue resistance was used: the time required for units to reach 50 percent of their initial force. These values exhibited a wide range among the 6 FF units (Table 1), thereby suggesting that the time to half force is a useful index for bringing out variations in the force-reduction profile (Figure 1).

The time to half force values are compared to enzyme activities in Figure 2. The 5 typical (non-potentiating) FF units reveal a significant relation between this index of fatigue resistance and LDH activity. However, no correlation was detected between this index and either MDH activity (Figure 2) or βOAC activity (not shown). This finding is not surprising because the short (2 min) duration of the presently used fatigue test would seem more likely to require glycolytic than oxidative metabolism (cf. Hermansen, 1981; Holloszy and Coyle, 1984).

The inclusion in the regression analysis of the one unit which displayed marked potentiation would remove the correlation between the time-to-half-force values and LDH activity (Figure 2). This observation and the difference in force profiles (Figure 1) suggest that the fatigability of the potentiating unit was probably dependent upon factors other than the level of glycolytic enzymes. Excitation failure can be ruled out as the cause for the precipitous fall in force, because the EMG amplitude remained consistently high for the duration of the fatigue test.

Based upon these preliminary data, two inferences can be drawn, although these must remain provisional until the accumulation of additional data. First, an association may well exist for non-potentiating FF units between the activity of glycolytic enzymes and fatigue resistance, as

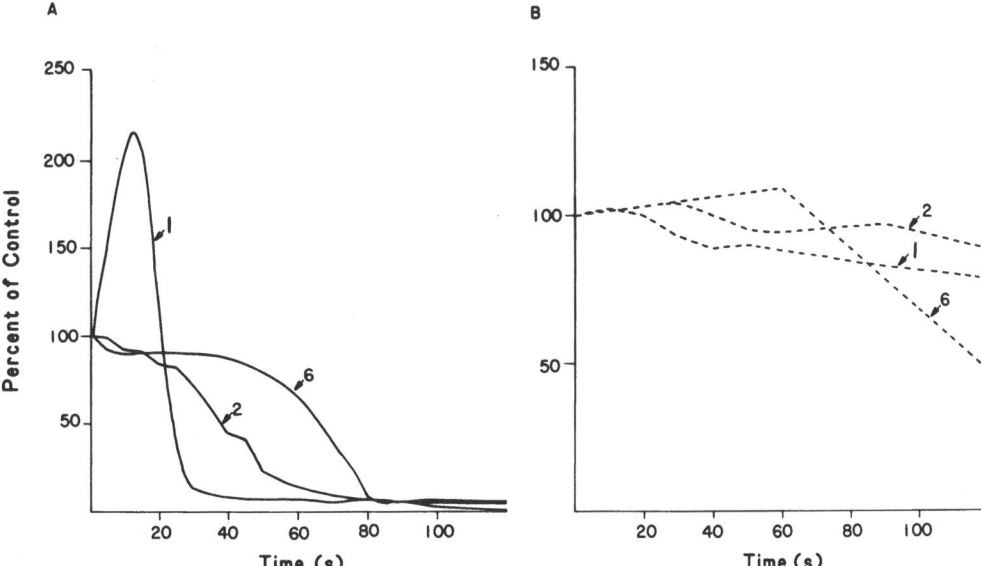

Fig. 1. Force and EMG profiles of single FF motor units during a standard
fatigue test. Each graph shows force (A; solid lines) and EMG (B;
dashed lines) as percentages of initial values plotted as a
function of time from the beginning of the fatigue test. Forces
shown are peak values during representative 330 ms, 40 Hz stimulus
trains throughout the 2 min test. EMG values are averaged peak-
to-peak values of the 13 action potentials of representative
trains. One unit (no.1; same as in Table 1) exhibited a substantial potentiation followed by a rapid decline in force. The
other 2 units (nos. 2 and 6, also same as in Table 1) showed
little force potentiation. These latter units had the shortest
(no.2; 38 s) and longest (no.6; 67 s) times required for a force
reduction to 50% of control values. Note that the EMG amplitude
of all 3 units was far less affected than the force throughout the
fatigue test.

measured using the stimulus paradigm of the presently used 2 min fatigue
test. Second, the absence of associations in the case of the potentiating
unit suggests that the enzyme activities in metabolic pathways in general
may not be the determining factor in fatigue resistance for all FF units
during the presently used tests. This inference must accommodate the fact
that the stimulus paradigm of the present test induced glycogen-depletion
in both the potentiating and non-potentiating units examined in this study.
What remains unknown, in this and all previous glycogen-depletion studies,
is the time course of the depletion process.

A dissociation of fatigue resistance and metabolic capacity indicates
a possible role for impaired excitation-contraction coupling (i.e., beyond
the excitation itself) during some experiemntal fatigue tests. This has
been reported recently, particularly for human subjects during "low-
frequency" (< 50 Hz) activation of their muscles (for review: Edwards,
1982). Similarly, it has been reported that FF, FI and many FR units in
another cat hindlimb muscle (peroneus tertius) are prone to a "delayed
fatigue" during the same fatigue test as used in the present study. This
fatigue was attributed to a "temporary failure of excitation-contraction
coupling" (Jami et al., 1983).

Table 1. Fatigue Resistance and Selected Enzyme Activities of FF Motor Units

	Fatigue indices*		Enzyme activities (mol/kg dry weight/hr)		
Unit no.	F_2'/F_0'	$t_{\frac{1}{2}}$ (s)	LDH	MDH	βOAC
1	0.05	25	312 ± 11	6.4 ± 0.4	2.6 ± 0.3
2	0.05	38	160 ± 7	4.6 ± 0.2	1.4 ± 0.1
3	0.05	43	234 ± 6	3.3 ± 0.2	1.4 ± 0.1
4	0.04	65	255 ± 16	5.2 ± 0.3	2.0 ± 0.3
5	0.03	66	251 ± 10	3.1 ± 0.2	1.4 ± 0.1
6	0.01	67	294 ± 6	4.0 ± 0.2	1.3 ± 0.1

*Fatigue resistance assessed in response to application of 330 ms, 40 Hz stimulus trains at a rate of 1 train/s. Fatigue indices calculated as ratio of peak force at 2 min of stimulation to that at start of stimulation (F_2'/F_0') and as time to reach 50% of initial force ($t_{\frac{1}{2}}$).

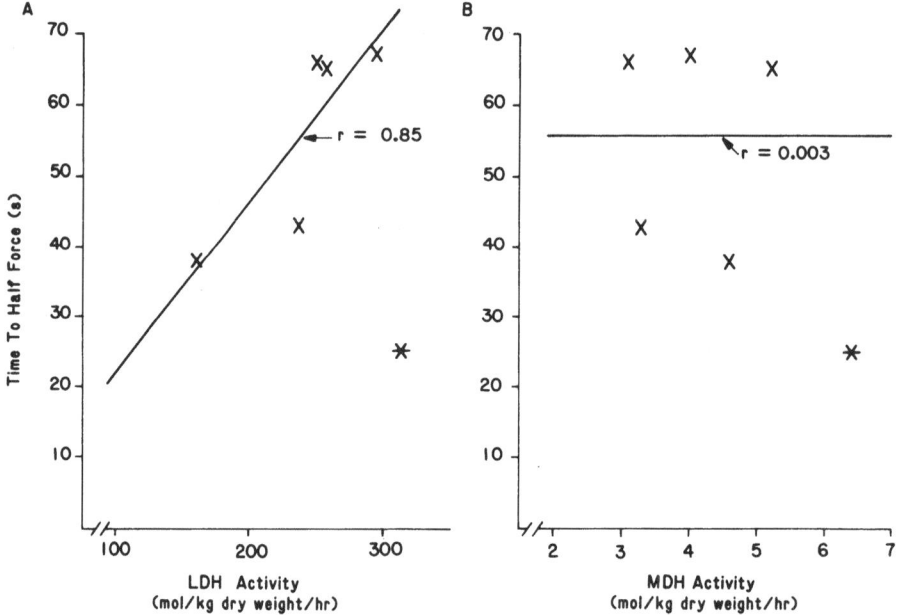

Fig. 2. Relationships between enzyme activities and fatigue resistance. The physiological index of fatigue resistance ($T_{\frac{1}{2}}$) was the time to reach 50% of initial force during a standard 2 min fatigue test. It is plotted against the activity of LDH (A) and MDH (B) of muscle fibers from the 6 FF motor units (same as in Table 1). The regression lines were calculated excluding the one unit (asterisk; no.1 in Table 1) which displayed marked potentiation. The correlation between $t_{\frac{1}{2}}$ and LDH activity was significant (r = 0.85, p<0.05). No correlation was found between $t_{\frac{1}{2}}$ and either MDH activity (r = 0.003, p>0.40) or βOAC activity (r = 0.28; p>0.25; not shown).

The presently used fatigue test has proven of particular value for the classification of motor units in cat hindlimb and now forelimb muscles (for review: Burke, 1981; Botterman et al., 1985). However, if the goal is to test for relationships between physiological and biochemical aspects of motor-unit fatigability, then the stimulus paradigm and duration of this test seem inappropriate for FF and possibly other motor-unit types. This issue requires further investigation, using techniques which quantitate the EMG-force relationship of motor units during fatigue tests, and which also provide a biochemical analysis of the units' constituent muscle fibers.

Acknowledgements

This work was supported by U.S.P.H.S. grants NS 18387 (to P.M.N.), NS 20544 (to D.G.S.) and HL 07249 (to the Department of Physiology), a grant from the Muscular Dystrophy Association (to P.M.N.), and by awards from the Bulgarian and U.S. Academies of Sciences (to T.M.H. and D.G.S.). We would like to thank L. Solanki, J. Park, P. Pierce, L. L. Rankin, K. Volz and Dr S. Vanden Noven for their assistance.

REFERENCES

Botterman, B. R., Iwamoto, G. A., and Gonyea, W. J., 1985, Classification of motor units in flexor carpi radialis muscle of the cat, J. Neurophysiol., 54:676.

Burke, R. E., 1981, Motor units: Anatomy, physiology and functional organization, in: "Handbook of Physiology, Section 1, Vol. II, The Nervous System: Motor Control, Part 1", V. B. Brooks, ed., Am. Physiol. Soc., Bethesda.

Burke, R. E., Levine, D. N., Tsairis, P., and Zajac, F. E., III, 1973, Physiological types and histochemical profiles in motor units of the cat gastrocnemius, J.Physiol.(London), 234:723.

Edstrom, L., and Kugelberg, E., 1968, Histochemical composition, distribution of fibers and fatigability of single motor units, J.Neurol. Neurosurg.Psychiat., 31:424.

Edwards, R. H. T., 1982, Weakness and fatigue of skeletal muscles, Adv. Med., 18:100.

Hermansen, L., 1981, Effect of metabolic changes in force generation in skeletal muscle during maximal exertion, in: "Human Muscle Fatigue: Physiological Mechanisms", R. Porter and J. Whelan, eds., Pitman, London.

Holloszy, J. O., and Coyle, E. F., 1984, Adaptations of skeletal muscle to endurance exercise and their metabolic consequences, J.Appl. Physiol.:Respirat.Environ.Exercise Physiol., 56:831.

Jami, L., Murthy, K. S. K., Petit, J., and Zytnicki, D., 1983, After-effects of repetitive stimulation at low frequency on fast-contracting motor units of cat muscle, J.Physiol.(London), 340:129.

Lowry, D. H., and Passoneau, J. V., 1972, "A Flexible System of Enzymatic Analysis", Academic, New York.

Nemeth, P. M., Pette, D., and Vrbova, G., 1981, Comparison of enzyme activities among single muscle fibers within defined motor units, J.Physiol.(London), 311:489.

Nemeth, P. M., Solanki, L., Gordon, D. A., Hamm, T. M., Reinking, R. M., and Stuart, D. G., 1985, Uniformity of metabolic enzymes within individual motor units, J.Neurosci., in press.

SECTION II
REFLEX CONTROL OF MOVEMENTS

DEVELOPMENT OF CUTANEOUS REFLEXES IN

THE UPPER LIMB DURING MAN ONTOGENESIS

V. Gatev, M. Stefanova-Uzunova, and L. Stamatova

Department of Developmental Physiology
Research Institute of Pediatrics
Sofia, Bulgaria

The cutaneous reflexes evoked by electrical stimuli have several electromyographic components in man. Collins et al. (1960) described two reflex responses. They accepted that the first of them is triggered by group second afferents, which evoked tactile sensation, while the second one is triggered by the activation of group third afferents, which evoked painful sensation. Hugon (1973) studied in detail these two cutaneous reflex responses in man. Recently Jenner and Stephens (1982) described triphasic modulation of the cutaneous reflex responses in man, the first and third-excitatory and the second-inhibitory. They presented evidence that the first component is spinal in origin, while the third one is supraspinal, most probably – transcortical.

Little information is available on the developmental mechanisms of cutaneous reflexes in children. Vecchierini-Blineau and Guiheneuc (1982) recorded the same two reflex responses in children, as they were described in adults by Hugon (1973). Issler and Stephens (1983), using averaged EMG recorded reflex responses by observing the modulation in ongoing muscle electrical activity produced by cutaneous stimulus, established in infants only short latency excitatory modulation. In children two years of age and in older they recorded short and long latency excitatory modulations. One year later using individual EMG we described three cutaneous reflex responses in leg and arm muscles of infants and small children (Gatev et al., 1984). In the present study we examined in detail the development of the arm cutaneous reflexes in man ontogenesis.

We studied normal children from birth till six years of age and adults. The upper limb was stimulated with ring electrodes. The cathode was placed around the fifth finger and the anode around the second one. The pulses were rectangular waves of 0.5 ms duration with frequency of 600 Hz, for 7 ms. The stimulus intensity was increased up to twice the threshold value. The reflex responses were recorded with bipolar electrodes, placed over flexor carpi ulnaris muscle in belly-tendon position. In some cases electrical activity was recorded from superficial extensor muscle group of the forearm. The latencies of reflex responses were measured from the beginning of stimulus artefact to the onset of reflex response.

In newborns, during the first month of life, only one, short latency response was recorded (Figure 1a). It is synchronious biphasic potential with negative first phase. After ipsilateral stimulation the short reflex response was expressed in flexor, as well as in extensor muscles. The short reflex response was not established following contralateral stimulation (Figure 1b).

In children aged from 1 month till 3 years we recorded three reflex responses: R_1 – short latency, R_2 – early long latency and R_3 – late long latency (Figure 2a). The latency of R_1 varied from 15.6 to 17.1 ms and was almost the same in 1-month, 1-year and 3-year-old children (Table 1). In 1-year and 3-year-old children the latency was about 40 ms for R_2 and 110 ms for R_3. The amplitude of R_1 diminished with age (630 μV in 1-month-olds, 215 μV in 1-year-olds and 161 μV in 3-year-olds). The two long latency responses were polyphasic, sometimes well separated and sometimes fused. Following ipsilateral stimulation all the three reflex responses were recorded in flexor as well as in extensor muscles. After contralateral stimulation we recorded only the long latency responses, both in flexor (Figure 2b) and in extensor muscles.

In order to clarify the origin of the short latency response we measured the length of the spinal pathway and its sensory and motor conduction velocities (Figure 3). The pathway was measured from the stimulating electrode to the skin overlying C_7 spinous process and from that point to the recording electrodes. The predicted latency was compared with the established one. No significant difference was found between them. This coincidence supports the spinal hypothesis for the short latency response. The latencies of all three reflex responses are almost equal in 1-month, 1-year and 3-year-old children (see the Table). This isolatency

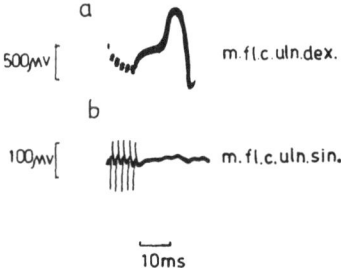

Fig. 1.   Short latency response following ipsilateral stimulation of the right hand (a) and absense of the same response in the left limb, contralateral to the stimulation (b).   Child aged 20 days.

Table 1.   Latency of Cutaneous Reflex Responses in Flexor Carpi Ulnaris

Age	R_1		R_2		R_3	
	n	$\bar{x} \pm s$	n	$\bar{x} \pm s$	n	$\bar{x} \pm s$
1-month (12)	12	17.1 ± 1.0	–	–	–	–
1-year (11)	11	15.6 ± 0.8	11	36.1 ± 7.9	11	109.1 ± 22.2
3-year (10)	8	16.0 ± 1.2	8	44.2 ± 6.5	10	107.0 ± 28.3

R_1 = short latency response; R_2 – early long latency response; R_3 – late long latency response; n – number of children in which reflex responses were obtained; $\bar{x}$ – mean; s – standard deviation; numbers in brackets indicate number of examined children.

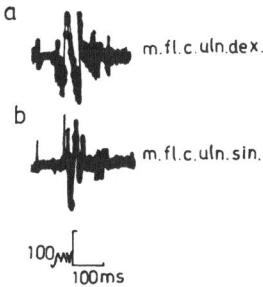

Fig. 2. Short and long latency responses following ipsilateral stimulation of the right hand (a) and long latency responses in the left limb (b). Child aged 2 years 6 months.

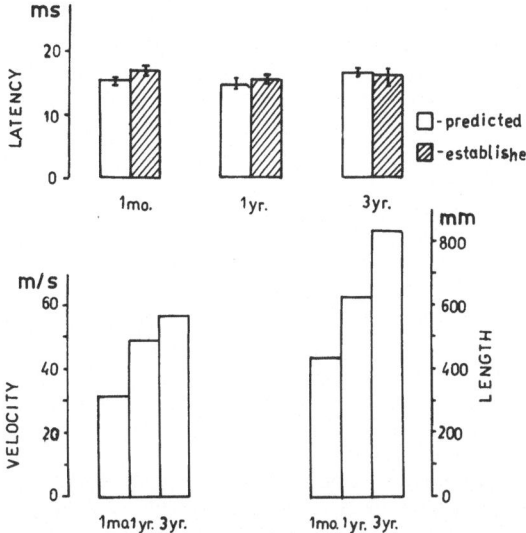

Fig. 3. Predicted and established short latency responses in flexor carpi ulnaris.

during the first three years of life may be explained with the fact that during this age period the increasing of conduction velocity is proportional to the lengthening of the neural pathway. After the third year the conduction velocity almost does not increase. As the length of the neural pathway increases twice in adults, the latency of the reflex responses also increases twice in them.

Our early long reflex response corresponds in latency to the first tactile response in adults (Hugon, 1973) and in children (Vecchierini-Blineau and Guiheneuc, 1982), and also to the second excitatory modulation described by Jenner and Stephens (1983) for which they accept transcortical pathway. Our late long reflex response corresponds to the second nociceptive response, described by the authors mentioned above. It is difficult to decide if this long latency response depends only on the smaller conduction velocity of the afferent pathway or/and on the longer central delay.

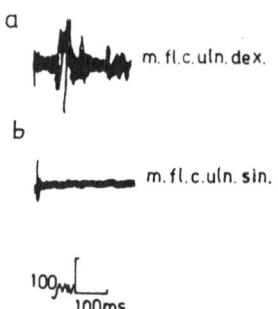

a   m.fl.c.uln.dex.

b   m.fl.c.uln.sin.

100μ͜V 100ms

Fig. 4. Long latency responses following ipsilateral stimulation of the right hand (a) and absense of the reflex responses in the left limb (b). Adult aged 26 years.

The short latency response gradually disappears in children from 3 to 6 years of age. In adults the short latency response was never found but the long latency responses were recorded in flexor (Figure 4a), as well as in extensor muscles following ipsi- and contralateral stimulation. In some adults the long latency responses were absent contralaterally (Figure 4b).

Summarizing the results from the present study we suppose that three stages in the development of cutaneous reflexes during man postnatal onto-genesis may be described.

The first stage begins from birth and terminates at the end of the first month of life. During this period only the short latency response can be recorded. This response was not found in the limb contralateral to the stimulation. There is some evidence that the short latency response is spinal in origin.

The second stage begins from the second month of life and ends at the third year. During this stage the short and the two long latency responses were recorded also in the limb contralateral to the stimulation. It is suggested that the appearance of the early long latency response shows that the corticospinal pathway begins to function.

The third ontogenetic stage of the postnatal development of cutaneous reflexes begins between three and six years of age and continues in adults. During this stage the short latency response disappears and only the long latency responses can be recorded. It is suggested that the disappearance of the short latency response is caused by the corticospinal facilitatory influence on the inhibitory pathways, which suppresses the spinal activity. The contralateral reflex response diminishes with age and in adults may be absent.

REFERENCES

Collins, W. F., Nulsen, F. E., and Randt, C. T., 1960, Relation of periph-
    eral nerve fiber size and sensation in man, Arch.Neurol.(Chic.),
    3:381.
Gatev, V., Uzunova, M., and Stamatova, L., 1984, An electrophysiological
    study of tactile and nociceptive cutaneous reflexes in children, in:
    "Pain", R. Rizzi and M. Visentin, eds., Piccin/Butterworths, Padua,
    p.239.

Hugon, M., 1973, Exteroceptive reflexes to stimulation of the sural nerve in normal man, in: "New Developments in Electromyography and Clinical Neurophysiology", J. E. Desmedt, ed., Karger, Basel, 3:713.

Issler, H., and Stephens, J. A., 1983, The maturation of cutaneous reflexes studied in the upper limb in man, J.Physiol.(London), 335:643.

Jenner, J. R., and Stephens, J. A., 1982, Cutaneous reflex responses and their nervous pathways studied in man, J.Physiol.(London), 333:405.

Vecchierini-Blineau, M. F., and Guiheneuc, P., 1982, Lower limb cutaneous polysynaptic reflex in the child, according to age and state of waking or sleeping, J.Neurol.Neurosurg.Psychiatr., 45:531.

M_2—A LONG LATENCY SPINAL REFLEX

DUE TO SKIN AFFERENTS IN MAN

M. Shahani, O. C. J. Lippold*, K. Darton**, and U. Shahani***

E.C.I. Institute of Electrophysiology for Fundamental and
Applied Research, Bombay, India
*Dept. of Human Physiology, Royal Hollaway College, Egham, U.K
**Dept. of Physiology and ***Dept. of Anatomy, University
College London, London, U.K.

A passive displacement of a limb when at rest is known to result in a
monosynaptic reflex. This is attributed to the excitation of Gr.IA afferents. Hammond[7] and later Marsden et al.[10,11,12] demonstrated a second
response (first being short latency monosynaptic) occurring at a long
latency when a perturbation was applied to a part of the limb which was
held in a position by isometric contraction of a muscle. On the basis of
calculating the latency of this second response, it was suggested to be
transcortical. A new terminology was suggested calling the first response
as M_1, the second response as M_2 and third very late response as M3[8,9].
Hagbarth[6] et al., questioned M_2 being a transcortical response on the
basis of recording spindle afferents discharges; they demonstrated that
when a muscle which is in contraction is stretched, the spindles seem to
discharge in an oscillatory manner. Matthews[13] on the other hand argued
that M_2 could be attributed to Gr.II afferents.

The authors decided to do some experiments which were carefully
designed in such a way as to avoid as far as possible the assumptions made
in the previous experiments. First dorsal interossei muscle was chosen,
which incidentally is supplied by the ulnar nerve (carrying efferent axons,
as well as afferent fibers from spindles) while the skin covering the index
finger (the part to be perturbed) is supplied by the median nerve.

MATERIALS AND METHOD

Several different experiments were carried out in normal healthy
volunteers, both male and female. Surface electrodes were used for the
purpose of recording from the first dorsal interossei muscle. The electromyographic signals were rectified and averaged (minimum 64 sweeps were
averaged); the same were displayed on an oscilloscope and later recorded
using an X-Y plotter. While the experiment was on, the subjects got a
visual feedback from a meter which showed the needle deflection in proportion to integrated EMG signal. Details of the technique used have been
previously described[1].

In the initial standard experiments, subjects were asked to rest their
hand on a platform while producing abduction of the index finger (asometric

contraction of first dorsal interossei muscle). Perturbance was produced
by a prod hitting the lateral border of the index finger at the level of
distal phalanx.

Keeping all the arrangements same as stated earlier, a prod was
applied to the medial side of the index finger, thus pushing the index
finger in the direction of abduction. In the other experiment, the hand
and arm were cooled with the prod being applied on the lateral border as in
the first set of experiments (stretching first dorsal interossei muscle).
Complete anesthesia over the index finger was achieved by applying tourniquet type pressure with tightly tied rubber bands just distal to the
metacarpophalangeal joint of the index finger; and the standard experiments
were carried out.

In another series of experiments, skin over the distal phalanx of the
index finger was stimulated while the first dorsal interossei was in isometric contraction. Electrical stimulation was also applied to the median
nerve at wrist, and then at elbow in another series of experiments.

Standard experiments were also performed in the foot using abductor
hallucis muscle for the studies.

RESULTS

In the standard experiments when prod was applied to displace the
index finger towards abduction, the first two bursts of electromyographic
activity (M_1 and M_2) were noticed at the mean latencies of 32.4 (SD 2.4 ms)
and 55.1 ms (SD 11.5 ms). A third burst of EMG activity was observed at
latencies longer than 100 ms (Figure 1).

In experiments involving prodding the index finger on the medial side
which in effect tended to shorten the muscle rather than stretch it, the
initial EMG burst was obtained at a latency compatible with M_2; there was
no M_1 (Figure 2).

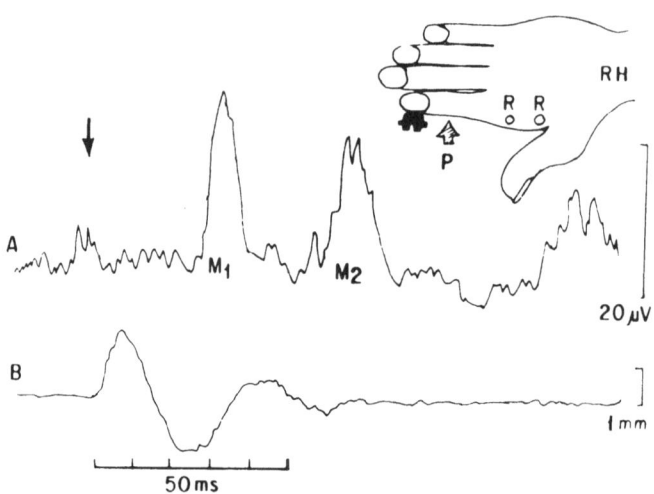

Fig. 1. 1st dorsal interosseus muscle in isometric contraction. M_1, M_2
responses on prodding lateral border of index finger (stretching
of the muscle).

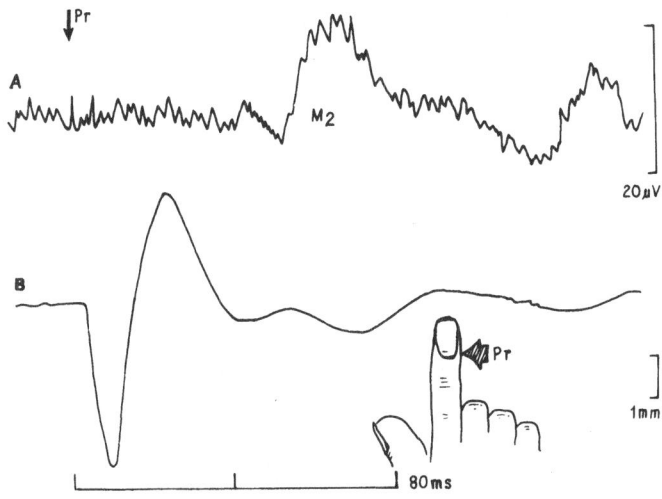

Fig. 2. 1st dorsal interosseus muscle in isometric contraction.
M_1 absent, M_2 present on prodding medial border of index finger
(no stretching of the muscle).

When an arm was cooled in the standard experiments, M_1 and M_2 were
obtained at almost equally delayed latencies (about 10 ms). This strongly
suggested that the afferents responsible for M_1 as well as M_2 are almost of
equal diameter and have similar conduction velocities. If M_2 were due to
Gr.II spindle afferents, the shift in the latency for M_2 would have had to
be greater. When a complete block was produced in the index finger (the
first dorsal interossei muscle lies proximal) by using tourniquet pressure
with rubber bands, M_2 was completely abolished, while M_1 was present
(Figure 3). This clearly demonstrated that M_2 was a response to cutaneous
afferent input.

There still remained the possibility that M_2 could be due to joint
afferents. In the next series of experiments when the skin over the distal
phalanx of the index finger was electrically stimulated, with first dorsal
interossei in isometric contraction, EMG burst was obtained at a latency
compatible with the latency of M_2 in the standard experiments.

When electrical stimulation was applied to the median nerve at the
wrist and then at the elbow, with first dorsal interossei in isometric
contraction, the EMG bursts were seen at suitable reduced latencies, as the
afferent pathway was reduced. By this method, conduction velocity of the
afferents was calculated, which was found to be approximately 50 m/s. It
must be noted that the median nerve does not carry the spindle afferents
from the first dorsal interossei muscle.

On doing the standard experiment of stretching the muscle with a prod,
in the case of abductor hallucis muscle in the foot, two early EMG bursts
(M_1 and M_2) were obtained at the latencies of 39.4 ms (SD 2.6 ms) and
66.3 ms (SD 2.9 ms). M_1-M_2 interval in the case of a muscle of the foot
was found to be about 27 ms, while the same in the case of first dorsal
interossei muscle in the hand was about 23 ms. If it was to be assumed
that M_2 response involved a transcortical loop, the pathway in the case of
a foot muscle would involve additional conduction time both ways from the

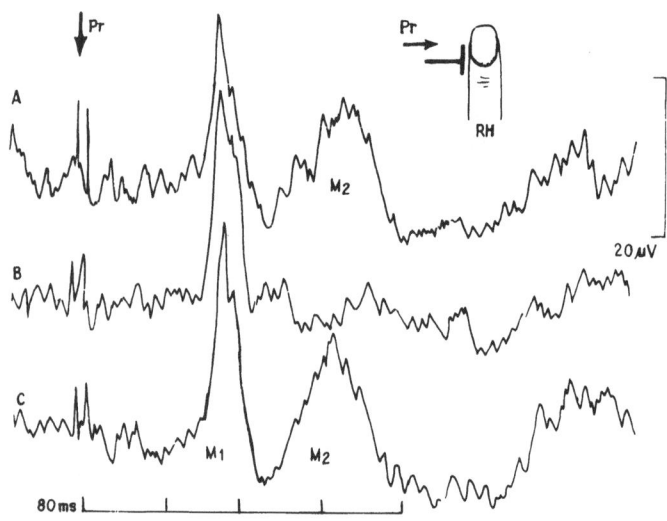

Fig. 3. 1st dorsal interosseus muscle in isometric contraction. Prodding
lateral border of index finger (stretching the muscle). M_2 absent
on blocking index finger nerves.

lumbar cord to the spinal cord (a distance over 25 cm in an adult); this
additional delay may be well over 15 ms (calculating conduction velocity at
50 m/s). As against this estimation, the M_1-M_2 interval in the case of a
foot muscle is just longer by about 4 ms than that for a muscle of the
hand.

DISCUSSION

The early experiments, perturbing a thumb or hand resulting in the
stretch of a muscle which was already in isometric contraction produced
three bursts of EMG activity. The very method involved stimulation of
various other afferents like cutaneous and joint afferents etc., besides
Gr.IA and Gr.II fibers from the muscle spindle; it was quite tempting for
the experimentors to assume that the second and third responses were due to
transcortical loops, as simultaneously some of the physiologists[2,3,4,5]
who were engaged in the study of motor cortex had suggested that motor
cortex should be doing something to handle Gr.IA information that reached
the sensory motor cortex.

The failure to abolish M_2 with anesthesia of distal parts as reported
in literature could be attributed to the design of experiments where the
force of perturbance was perhaps so large as to excite in addition the
mechano-receptors in the skin far away from the site of the contact of the
perturbing device, thus exciting cutaneous afferents which were lying
proximal to the anesthetized skin. In the experiments reported here, the
force applied with the prod was not so large, and the same was applied to
the distal phalanx of the index finger; both the factors made it doublely
sure that when the index finger was blocked completely, there was no excitation of cutaneous afferents at all; this resulted in the abolishing of
M_2 completely. That M_2 was due to cutaneous afferents was conclusively
proved when it could be obtained at exactly the same latency as in the
perturbing experiments, when the same area of the skin was electrically

stimulated. By further experiments, when the median nerve (which supplied the skin in the index finger) was stimulated at wrist and then at elbow, M_2 was obtained at proportionately shorter latencies which helped the authors to calculate the conduction velocity of the cutaneous afferents involved to 50 m/s. The choice of first dorsal interossei muscle made it possible to conduct these experiments as this muscle is supplied by ulnar nerve, while the cutaneous area involved is supplied by the median nerve.

In order to check whether M_2 response was transcortical or spinal, it was decided to elicit these responses from abductor hallucis muscle in the foot. The time interval between M_1 and M_2 was more or less the same in both the cases, i.e., finger and toe. If M_2 responses were to involve a transcortical loop, the M_1-M_2 interval in the case of muscle of the foot would have had to be longer by about 15 ms or so (conduction time along the spinal cord from the lumbar cord to the cervical cord and back). It is therefore suggested that M_2 response does not involve a long transcortical loop.

M_2 response due to cutaneous afferents is produced at spinal level when the central excitatory state of the concerned motor neuronal pool is already raised by corticospinal drive. It could be hypothesized that the physiological significance of this M_2 response may be to restore or retain ongoing activity in the concerned muscle. It is interesting to report (unpublished data) that when the median nerve was stimulated at the wrist or there was perturbance produced by applying a prod on the dorsal or ventral surfaces of the wrist, M_2 could be elicited from triceps or biceps muscles whichever was already held in isometric contraction. Similar results in the case of a cat in locomotion have been reported[5a]. However, no response could be obtained from either biceps or triceps muscles if the subject was asked to keep the elbow stiff by producing a contraction of the biceps and triceps muscles. In view of the current evidence, it seems fair to postulate that M_2 response which is due to cutaneous afferents, is occurring at the spinal level and perhaps subserves the physiological function of sustaining the ongoing program of the motor activity.

REFERENCES

1. K. Darton, O. C. J. Lippold, M. Shahani, and U. Shahani, Long latency spinal reflexes in humans, J.Neurophysiol., 53(6):1605-1618 (June 1985).
2. E. V. Evarts, Motor cortex reflexes associated with learned movement, Science, 179:501-503 (1973).
3. E. V. Evarts and R. Granit, Relations of reflexes and intended movements, in: "Understanding the Stretch Reflex, Progress in Brain Research", S. Homma, ed., 44:1-14, Elsevier, Amsterdam (1976).
4. E. V. Evarts and J. Tanji, Reflex and intended response in motor cortex pyramidal tract neurones of monkey, J.Neurophysiol., 39:1069-1089 (1976).
5. E. V. Evarts and W. J. Vaughan, Intended arm movements in response to externally produced arm displacements in man, in: "Cerebral Motor Control in Man: Long Loop Mechanisms, Progress in Clinical Neurophysiology", J. E. Desmedt, ed., 4:178-192, Karger, Basel (1978).
5a H. Forssberg, S. Grillner, S. Rossignol, and P. Wallen, Phasic control of reflexes during locomotion in vertebrates, in: "Neurol Control of Locomotion", R. M. Herman et al., eds., pp. 647-676, Plenum Press, New York (1976).
6. K. E. Hagbarth, J. V. Hagglund, E. V. Wallin, and R. R. Young, Grouped spindle and electromyographic responses to abrupt wrist extension movements in man, J.Physiol., 312:81-96 (1981).

7. P. H. Hammond, Involuntary activity in biceps following the sudden application of velocity to the abducted forearm, <u>J.Physiol.</u>, 127:23–25P (1965).

8. R. G. Lee and W. G. Tatton, Motor responses to sudden limb displacements in primates with specific CNS lesions and in human patients with motor system disorders, <u>Can.J.Neurol Sci.</u>, 2:285–293 (1975).

9. R. G. Lee and W. G. Tatton, Long loop reflexes in man: clinical applications, <u>in</u>: "Progr. Clin. Neurophysiol.", J. E. Desmedt, ed., 4:342–360, Karger, Basel (1978).

10. C. D. Marsden, P. A. Merton, and H. B. Morton, Servoaction in human voluntary movement, <u>Nature</u>, 238:140–143 (1972).

11. C. D. Marsden, P. A. Merton, and H. B. Morton, Servoaction in the human thumb, <u>J.Physiol.</u>, 257:1–44 (1976).

12. C. D. Marsden, P. A. Merton, and H. B. Morton, Stretch reflex and servoaction in a variety of human muscles, <u>J.Physiol.</u>, 259:531–560 (1976).

13. P. B. C. Matthews, Does the 'long latency' component of the human stretch reflex depend after all on spindle secondary afferents?, <u>J.Physiol.</u>, 341:16P (1983).

FACTORS WHICH MODIFY THE SHORT AND LONG LATENCY

COMPONENTS OF THE STRETCH REFLEX IN THE HUMAN FOREARM

R. G. Lee, R. Hayashi, and W. Becker

Department of Clinical Neurosciences
Faculty of Medicine, University of Calgary
Calgary, Alberta, Canada

INTRODUCTION

When sudden mechanical perturbations are applied at a joint, the muscle which is undergoing stretch exhibits a complex EMG response which includes both short latency and long latency components. The short latency component (M1) represents a spinal reflex mediated mainly by group IA muscle spindle afferents. The origin of the long latency component (M2) has been a topic of ongoing debate. Some investigators believe that it is mediated entirely or in part by a long loop transcortical pathway, while others argue that it can be accounted for entirely by spinal mechanisms. (For detailed reviews see Lee et al., 1983; Marsden et al., 1983.)

Recent studies have focussed on the types of receptors and peripheral afferent pathways which mediate the M1 and M2 components of the stretch reflex. Two major views have emerged from these studies. Hagbarth and his colleagues (1981) have proposed that M2 occurs as a result of repetitive bursts of activity from primary spindle endings. Their recordings have shown segmentation of the afferent discharge in IA fibers which could account for the segmentation of the EMG response. On the other hand, Matthews (1984) has recently presented experimental data suggesting that group II afferents from spindle secondary endings are responsible for the M2 response.

There are a number of factors which can modify afferent input from muscle stretch receptors. Some of these such as vibration and ischemia have different effects on group IA and group II spindle afferents. They also differ in the manner in which they modify the M1 and M2 components of the stretch reflex. By studying how these factors modify M1 and M2 we may gain additional insights concerning the afferent inputs which mediate these reflex components.

VIBRATION

Vibration is a powerful activator of spindle primary endings and IA afferents (Lance et al., 1973). Somewhat paradoxically, it also suppresses tendon jerks and H-reflexes (see Desmedt, 1983), probably due to increased activation of presynaptic inhibition of IA afferent terminals (Gillies et al., 1969).

If M1 and M2 are mediated by the same afferent pathways and the same spinal mechanisms, they should respond to vibration in a similar manner. Previous studies from our laboratory (Hendrie and Lee, 1978) and by others (Agarwal and Gottlieb, 1980) have shown that this is not the case. M1 is suppressed by vibration, but M2 is not affected. An example from a normal subject is shown in Figure 1. This illustrates rectified and averaged EMG activity from the wrist flexor muscles following sudden extension perturbations at the wrist produced by a torque motor. The subject was instructed to voluntarily oppose the displacement, a technique which consistently accentuates the M2 component. During the recording illustrated by the lower EMG trace in Figure 1, a commercial 100 Hz vibrator was held firmly over the wrist flexor tendons throughout the recording period. Note the marked suppression of M1 with no obvious change in M2.

These observations would be compatible with the proposal that M2 is mediated by group II afferents, since we know that these fibers are much less sensitive to vibration than IA afferents. The results from vibration studies do not, however, entirely exclude the possibility that M2 and M1 are both mediated by IA afferents. The afferent fibers which are responsible for M2 could form different connections in the spinal cord such that they were not subjected to the same amount of presynaptic inhibition associated with the application of vibration.

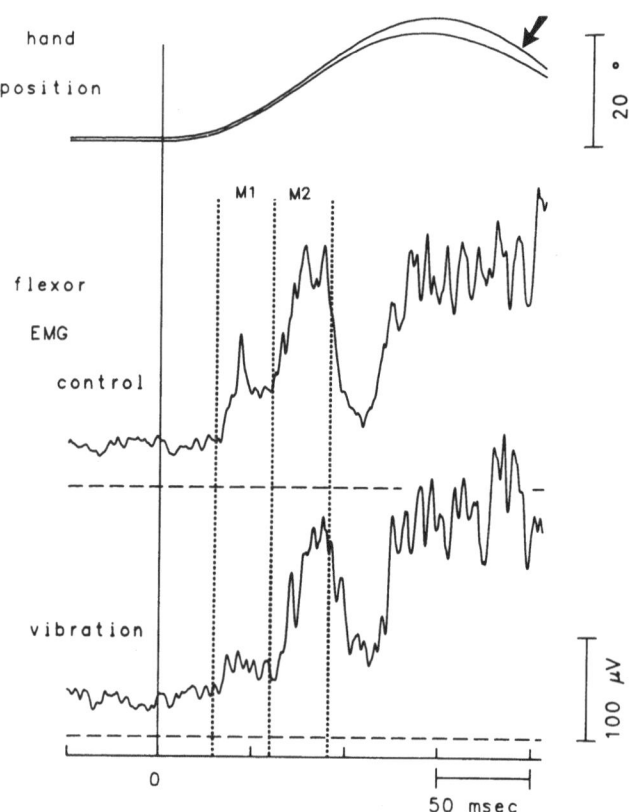

Fig. 1.   Effect of vibration on EMG responses to extension perturbations at the wrist. EMG traces represent an average of 10 responses recorded from wrist flexors. Note suppression of M1 during vibration. Corresponding position trace (arrow) shows greater displacement of wrist when M1 is suppressed.

ISCHEMIC NERVE BLOCK

   Since the rate at which ischemic nerve block develops varies according
to fiber size, ischemia provides another method for modifying the afferent
input resulting from muscle stretch. In 6 normal subjects we studied the
EMG responses in the wrist flexor muscles to extension perturbations at the
wrist joint. After initial control recordings were obtained, a blood
pressure cuff was placed around the upper arm and inflated to a pressure of
200 mm Hg. Responses to wrist perturbations were recorded at 4 minute
intervals until a complete nerve block occurred, usually 25-30 minutes
after inflation of the cuff.

   Results from this experiment are shown in Figure 2. Since the rate at
which the ischemic block developed varied slightly amongst the different
subjects, we have normalized the time scale to allow comparison of results
from all subjects. On this scale 100 represents the time at which the
amplitude of the M2 component has decreased to 15% of its control value.
The values on the ordinate represent integrated EMG activity for the M1
interval (30-60 ms after onset of perturbation) and the M2 interval (60-
90 ms). Note that M2 begins to decrease in size before M1 (at about 30% on
the normalized time scale) and remains consistently more suppressed than M1
throughout the period during which the ischemic block is developing.

   Suppression of these reflexes could occur as a result of blocking of
either afferent or efferent fibers. In a subsequent experiment we stimulated the median nerve in the axilla above the cuff and found that the motor

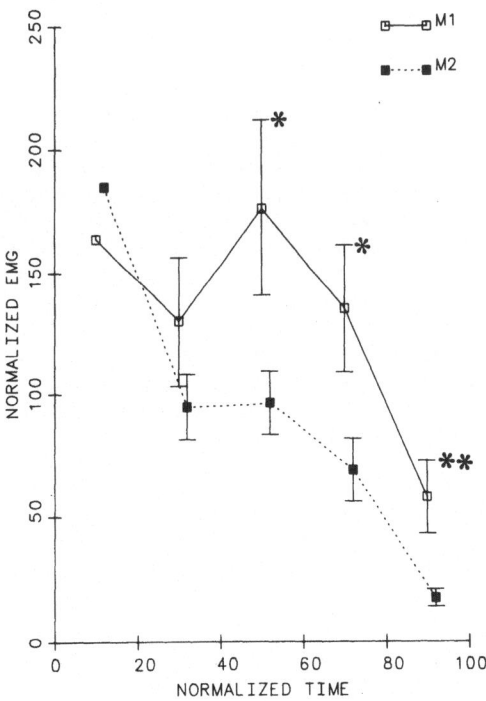

Fig. 2. Effect of ischemic nerve block on M1 and M2 components of the
         stretch reflex. Each point represents the mean EMG area ± 1SE.
         Time scale has been normalized to allow comparison between
         different subjects (see text). Note greater suppression of M2 as
         the ischemic block develops. (*p<0.05, **p<0.01).

response to median nerve stimulation was still preserved at a time when the tendon jerk from the forearm muscle was suppressed and also when sensation in the hand and forearm was diminished. This would suggest that suppression of M1 and M2, at least during the early stage of ischemia, occurs as a result of ischemic block of afferent fibers.

Why should M2 be affected differently from M1? If both reflex components were mediated by the same population of afferent fibers, we would expect them to be equally sensitive to ischemia. However, if M2 is mediated by group II spindle afferents as proposed by Matthews (1984) it should be suppressed earlier than M1 since small diameter fibers are more sensitive to the effects of ischemia than large fibers (Fox and Kenmore, 1967). One problem with this interpretation is that there is some uncertainty as to how much of the nerve block produced by a tourniquet or cuff is due to pure ischemia as opposed to mechanical compression of the nerve, a factor which we know affects large fibers earlier than small fibers.

STIMULATION OF CUTANEOUS AFFERENTS

Activation of cutaneous afferents produces a series of inhibitory and excitatory modulations of the tonic EMG activity associated with a steady voluntary contraction (Garnett and Stephens, 1980). The exact form of these changes depend on the site of stimulation and the muscle which is being activated. In subjects contracting the wrist flexors against a moderate load, stimulation of the digital nerves of the three middle fingers causes a prominent inhibition of tonic EMG activity beginning 39 ms after the stimulus and lasting approximately 30 ms.

By combining electrical stimulation with mechanical perturbations it is possible to compare the effects of a conditioning stimulus of cutaneous nerves on the M1 and M2 components of the stretch reflex. We have used this approach to investigate normal subjects and also a group of hemiplegic patients. The electrical stimulus consisted of a brief train (3 pulses of 0.2 ms duration at a frequency of 300 Hz) delivered simultaneously to the second, third, and fourth digits. The mechanical stimulus was the same as what has already been described - an extension perturbation at the wrist causing sudden stretch of the wrist flexors. The timing between the electrical and mechanical stimuli was varied so that the expected period of EMG inhibition resulting from the electrical stimulus coincided with either the M1 or M2 component of the stretch evoked EMG response.

Results from one normal subject are shown in Figure 3. Although both M1 and M2 are inhibited by activation of cutaneous afferents, the inhibitory effect is much greater on M2. This has been a constant finding in all normal subjects studied with this method.

To interpret these results we have to consider the mechanisms by which stimulation of cutaneous afferents can reduce motoneuron excitability. In the cat, cutaneous afferents, acting through an interneuron, excite Ib inhibitory interneurons, which in turn produce direct inhibition of motoneurons (Lundberg et al., 1977). If this pathway is also present in the human spinal cord, it would seem to be a logical candidate to mediate the inhibitory effects resulting from stimulation of digital nerves. But again we are left with the observation that M2 is affected differently from M1. This would be difficult to explain if M2 was merely a spinal reflex resulting from continuous or repetitive activation of the same pathways responsible for M1. However, as indicated previously there is strong evidence to support the concept that M2 is mediated, at least in part, by a long loop transcortical pathway. Ib inhibitory interneurons are facilitated by descending activity in the corticospinal tract (Illert et al., 1976). If

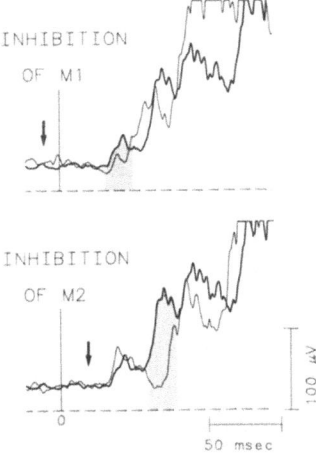

INHIBITION
OF M1

INHIBITION
OF M2

100 μV

0

50 msec

Fig. 3. Rectified and averaged EMG responses from the wrist flexors of a
normal subject. At time zero, indicated by the vertical line, an
extension perturbation of the wrist was produced by a torque
motor. At the times indicated by the arrows, a short train of
electrical stimuli was delivered to the three middle digits.
Shaded area represents the expected period of inhibition resulting
from electrical stimulation. Dark traces are the responses to
mechanical perturbations alone; light traces are responses to
combination of electrical and mechanical stimuli. Note that M2
(lower traces) is more inhibited by electrical stimulation than
M1.

the mechanical perturbation used in our experiments generated afferent
activity which travelled to cerebral cortex and back down to spinal cord,
it is conceivable that the Ib inhibitory interneuron might receive
additional excitation from this source at the same time it was being
activated by cutaneous afferents. The net result would be increased
inhibition of motoneurons at the time of the M2 response.

This concept receives some support from observations on patients with
hemiplegia resulting from infarcts of one cerebral hemisphere. We have
studied six hemiplegic patients using the same technique of conditioning
electrical stimulation of digital nerves combined with mechanical perturbations at the wrist. Pooled results are shown in Figure 4. In the clinically normal arm, the results were the same as what was observed in normal
subjects: M2 was significantly more inhibited than M1. However, in the
paretic arms inhibition of M1 and M2 was equal. This could be accounted
for by interruption of a transcortical reflex loop in the damaged cerebral
hemisphere. The additional facilitation of Ib inhibitory interneurons by
descending activity in the corticospinal tract would be reduced in this
situation.

OTHER FACTORS WHICH MODIFY THE M1 AND M2 COMPONENTS OF THE STRETCH REFLEX

Several other factors are capable of modifying the M1 and M2 components, either together or independently. These are summarized in Table 1.

The mechanical properties of the perturbation are important. It has
been shown that both M1 and M2 are graded responses which increase in a
linear manner as a function of the initial velocity of the imposed dis-

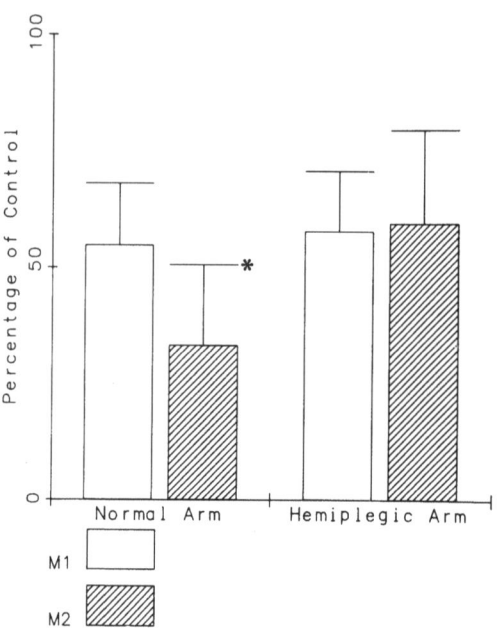

Fig. 4. Effect of electrical stimulation of digital nerves on EMG
responses to extension perturbations of the wrist in 6 hemiplegic
patients. Values shown represent means and standard errors for
area of M1 and M2 expressed as a percentage of control responses
recorded without electrical stimulation. M2 is more inhibited
than M1 in the normal arm (*p<0.01), but not in the paretic arm.

placement (Tatton et al., 1984). The M2 component is also very dependent
on the duration of the displacement (Lee and Tatton, 1982). Brief perturbations which are arrested prior to 40 ms after their onset produce only an
M1 response. This is similar to what is observed with the phasic stimulus
produced by a tendon tap. M2 appears only when the displacement is maintained for longer than 40 ms. One interpretation of this observation is
that M2 occurs as a result of convergent excitatory inputs to motoneurons
both from the periphery and from supraspinal centres which form part of a
long loop reflex pathway.

Volitional set or prior instruction to the subject has a marked
influence on the M2 component as noted originally by Hammon (1954). If the
subject is instructed to ignore the perturbation or to "let go", the M2
component is quite small. However, when the subject is told to "oppose"
the perturbation a well developed M2 response is seen (Lee and Tatton,
1975). It has been proposed that there is a gating mechanism, possibly at
the level of the sensorimotor cortex whereby feedback in the transcortical
loop is modulated to levels which are appropriate for the specific motor
task being performed.

Our understanding of the afferent pathways which generate M1 and M2 is
also helped by considering factors which do not modify these EMG responses.
The mechanical perturbations used to generate these responses activate
cutaneous and joint afferents as well as muscle afferents. However,
blocking cutaneous and joint afferents with local anesthetic does not
significantly alter either the M1 and M2 component, suggesting that these
responses occur primarily as a result of activation of muscle stretch
receptors (Bawa and McKenzie, 1981).

Table 1. Summary of Factors which Selectively Modify the M1 and M2
Components of the Stretch Reflex

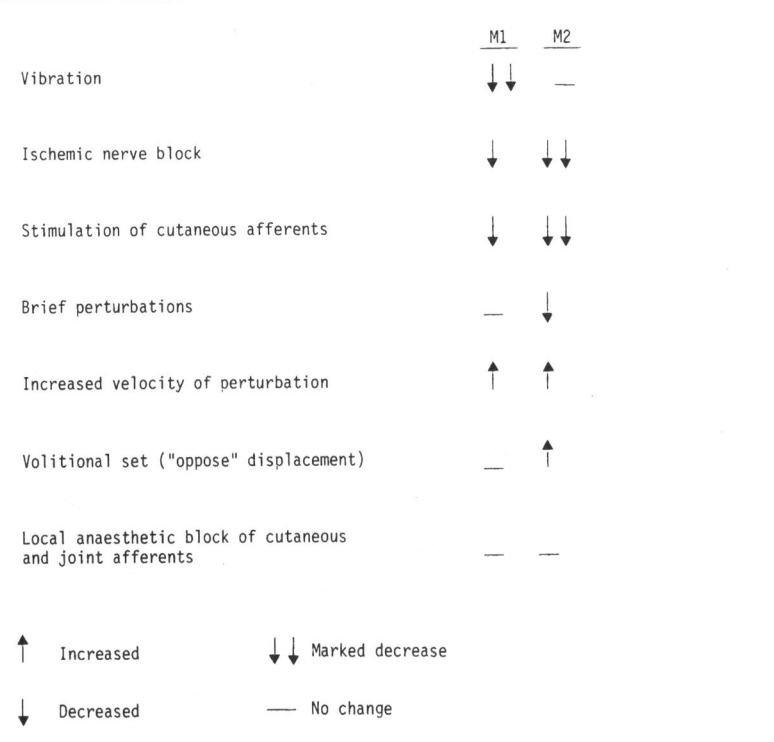

	M1	M2
Vibration	↓↓	—
Ischemic nerve block	↓	↓↓
Stimulation of cutaneous afferents	↓	↓↓
Brief perturbations	—	↓
Increased velocity of perturbation	↑	↑
Volitional set ("oppose" displacement)	—	↑
Local anaesthetic block of cutaneous and joint afferents	—	—

↑ Increased   ↓↓ Marked decrease

↓ Decreased   —— No change

CONCLUSIONS

It is apparent that M1 and M2 components of the stretch reflex are
differentially affected by several modifying factors. Some of these
observations are difficult to interpret if M2 results entirely from
activation of the same population of afferent fibers which mediate M1.
The results of the experiments with vibration and ischemic nerve block in
particular would be consistent with M2 being mediated by group II afferents
from muscle spindle secondary endings. Matthews (1984) has argued that
slow conduction in group II afferents is sufficient to account for the long
latency of M2 without postulating a long loop reflex pathway. However, in
our experience the M2 response in the wrist flexors begins approximately
60 ms following the onset of the perturbation. Considering time factors
alone, we believe that there is ample time for signals travelling in group
II afferents in the periphery to reach the cerebral cortex and return to
the spinal cord to generate an EMG response at this latency.

REFERENCES

Agarwal, G. C., and Gottlieb, G. L., 1980, Effect of vibration on the ankle
    reflex in man, Electroenceph.Clin.Neurophysiol.
Bawa, P., and McKenzie, D. C., 1981, Contribution of joint and cutaneous
    afferents to longer-latency reflexes in man, Brain Res.,
    211:185-189.
Bedingham, W., and Tatton, W. G., 1984, Dependence of EMG responses evoked
    by imposed wrist displacement on pre-existing activity in the
    stretched muscles, Can.J.Neurol.Sci., 11:272-280.

Desmedt, J. E., 1983, Mechanisms of vibration-induced inhibition or potentiation: tonic vibration reflex and vibration paradox in man, in: "Motor Control Mechanisms in Health and Disease", J. E. Desmedt, ed., pp. 671-683, Raven Press, New York.

Fox, J. L., and Kenmore, P. I., 1967, The effect of ischemia on nerve conduction, Exp.Neurol., 17:403-419.

Garnett, R., and Stephens, J. A., 1980, The reflex responses of single motor units in human first dorsal interrosseous muscles following cutaneous afferent stimulation, J.Physiol., 303:351-364.

Gillies, J. D., Lance, J. W., Neilson, P. D., and Tassinari, C. A., 1969, Recent inhibition of the monosynaptic reflex by vibration, J.Physiol., 205:329-339.

Hagbarth, K. E., Hagglund, J. V., Wallin, E. U., and Young, R. R., 1981, Grouped spindle and electromyographic responses to abrupt wrist extension movements in man, J.Physiol., 312:81-96.

Hammmond, P., 1954, Involuntary activity in biceps following a sudden application of velocity to the abducted forearm, J.Physiol., 127:23-25.

Hendrie, A., and Lee, R. G., 1978, Selective effects of vibration on human spindle and long-loop reflexes, Brain Res., 157:369-375.

Illert, M., Lundberg, A., and Tanaka, R., 1976, Integration in descending motor pathways controlling the forelimb in the cat, Exp.Brain Res., 26:521-540.

Lance, J. W., Burke, D., and Andrews, C. J., 1973, The reflex effects of muscle vibration. Studies of tendon jerk irradiation, and the tonic vibration reflex, in: "New Developments in Electromyography and Clinical Neurophysiology", J. E. Desmedt, ed., 3:444-462, Karger, Basel.

Lee, R. G., and Tatton, W. G., 1975, Motor responses to sudden limb displacements in primates with specific CNS lesions and in human patients with motor system disorders, Can.J.Neurol.Sci., 2:285-293.

Lee, R. G., Murphy, J. T., and Tatton, W. G., 1983, Long-latency myotatic reflexes in man: mechanisms, functional significance and changes in patients with Parkinson's Disease or hemiplegia, in: "Motor Control Mechanisms in Health and Disease", J. E. Desmedt, ed., pp. 489-508, Raven Press, New York.

Lundberg, A., Malgren, K., and Schomberg, E. D., 1977, Cutaneous facilitation of transmission and reflex pathways from Ib afferents to motoneurons, J.Physiol., 265:763-780.

Marsden, C. D., Rothwell, J. C., and Day, B. L., 1983, Long-latency automatic responses to muscle stretch in man: origin and function, in: "Motor Control Mechanisms in Health and Disease", J. E. Desmedt, ed., pp. 509-540, Raven Press, New York.

Matthews, P. B. C., 1984, Evidence from the use of vibration that the human long-latency stretch reflex depends upon spindle secondary afferents, J.Physiol., 348:383-415.

CHANGES IN STRETCH RESPONSES DUE TO HYPOTONIA

A. Struppler, H. Riescher, and L. Gerilovsky*

Department of Neurology
Technical University
Munich

Hypotonia may be clinically obvious under different conditions. In the lying position, hypotonia of the extremities is a result of decreased myotatic reflexes. In the upright position, altered supraspinal descending influences come into play. During isometric innervation hypotonia can be investigated by examining excursions of the limb produced by mechanical perturbations. When the subject tries to counteract the excursion of his limb segment, an overshooting compensation occurs.

Hypotonia can be caused by lesions at various levels in the somato-sensory afferent system (Table 1). In hypotonia of peripheral origin p.e. polyneuropathy-syndrome or in dorsal root lesions, like Tabes dorsalis, there are usually deficiencies in many somatosensory modalities, the so-called discriminative abilities and the tendon reflexes are abolished. If during the so-called differential block preferential gamma-axons con-comitantly with other small nerve fibers are blocked, the tendon reflex disappeared due to a loss of spindle drive. In dorsal column lesions, position sense as well as vibratory sense are diminished, the tendon reflexes, however, remain unchanged. In hypotonia of cerebellar origin the so-called epicritic sensibility as well as the phasic tendon reflexes remain unchanged, but there is a combination with ataxia. A special form of hypotonia, however, can be observed following small stereotaxic lesions on subthalamic or thalamic (VL) level.

Discrete stereotaxic lesions in the Nucleus ventrolateralis of the thalamus (VL) and in the subthalamus can abolish resting, postural and intention tremor. Concomitantly, rigidity as well as the tonic reflex excitability are decreased or even abolished. Reinforcement (Jendrassik manoeuver or mental drive) no longer evoke tremor or rigidity. The patient shows a postural hypotonia that can be compensated for by visual control. The rebound phenomenon (Stewart-Holmes), following sudden unloading of the muscle (isometrically activated by holding a light weight), is diminished. Motor force, rapid movement and phasic stretch reflexes, however, remain unchanged.

*Recipient of a A.v. Humboldt-Fellowship in 1984; present address: Central Laboratory of Biophysics, Bulg. Acad. of Sciences, Sofia, Bulgaria.

Table 1.

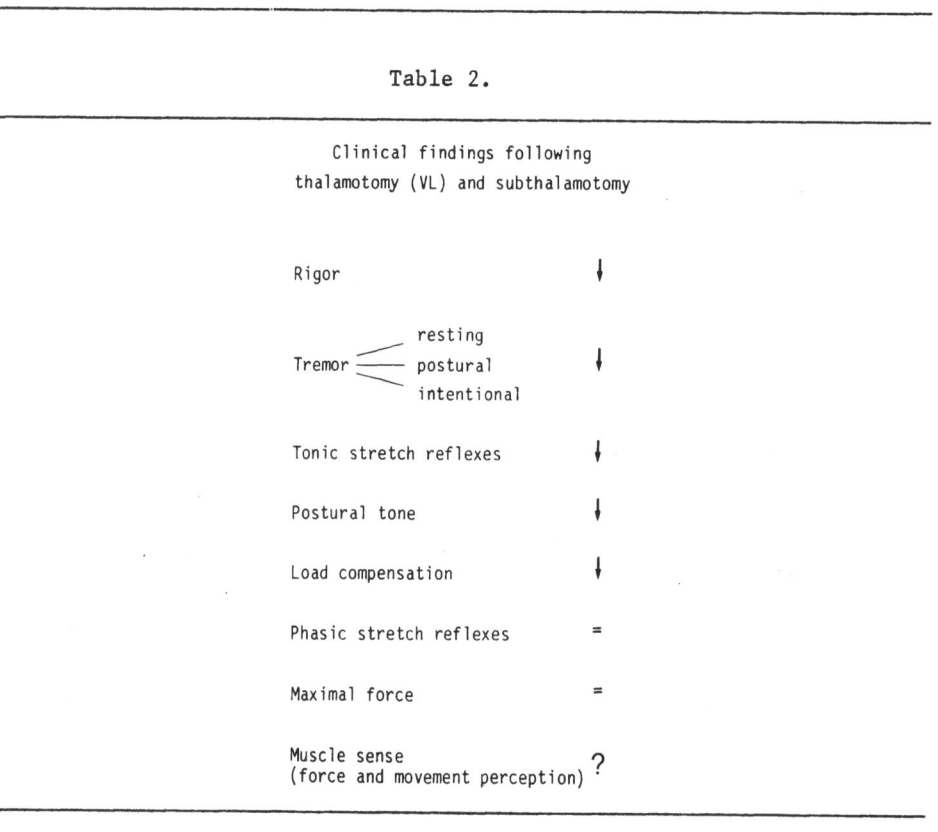

HYPOTONIA

CAN ARISE FOLLOWING:		PHASIC STRETCH REFLEX
1. DORSAL ROOT LESIONS	(SPINDLE AFFERENTS ↓)	↓
2. DIFFERENTIAL BLOCK	(GAMMA EFFERENTS ↓)	↓
3. DORSAL COLUMN LESIONS	(ASCENDING SPINAL AFFERENTS ↓)	NORMAL
4. CEREBELLAR LESIONS	(ALPHA-GAMMA- LINKAGE ↓)	NORMAL
5. THALAMOTOMY OR SUB- THALAMOTOMY	(ASCENDING MUSCLE AFFERENTS ↓?)	NORMAL

Table 2.

Clinical findings following
thalamotomy (VL) and subthalamotomy

Rigor	↓
Tremor — resting / postural / intentional	↓
Tonic stretch reflexes	↓
Postural tone	↓
Load compensation	↓
Phasic stretch reflexes	=
Maximal force	=
Muscle sense (force and movement perception)	?

If the lesion is small enough, there is no ataxia and no deficit of the so-called epicritic sensitivity, like perception of touch or joint movement. Evaluation of muscle force, however, seems to be disturbed.

The hypotonia of subthalamic origin seems to be for us the best model to investigate: how can sudden external perturbation be compensated in hypotonic states? How will the CNS react to sudden stretch under isometric conditions?

The flexor muscles of the forearm were investigated because they contribute to posture, particularly in the upright position. Moreover, these muscles are used predominantly for developing force and for adaptation for external perturbations in comparison to our finger muscles.

METHODS

Both forearms of the patient were fixed to the levers moved by 2 independently operating precision torque motors, which could perform constant torque from 0 to 6 Nm against the action of the forearm flexor muscles. Additionally, sudden torque pulses (0 to 6 Nm, risetime 5 ms, duration 1 s) could be applied. EMG, joint ankle (position) and force were recorded.

In parkinsonian patients there is an increased M2-component, as shown by Tatton and Lee (1975). Following stereotaxic lesions, M2 was clearly normalized, associated with a pronounced overshoot and an elongation of the elbow flexors (Lehmann-Horn et al., 1982).

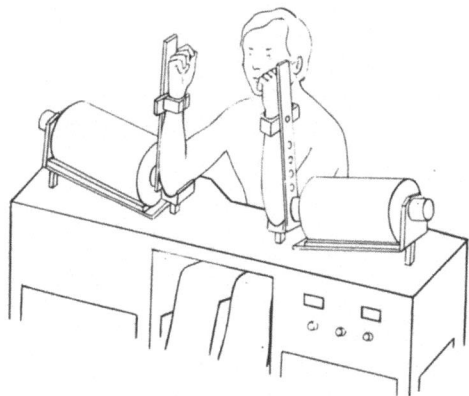

Fig. 1. Experimental set-up to investigate muscle response, when stretches are applied to the forearm.

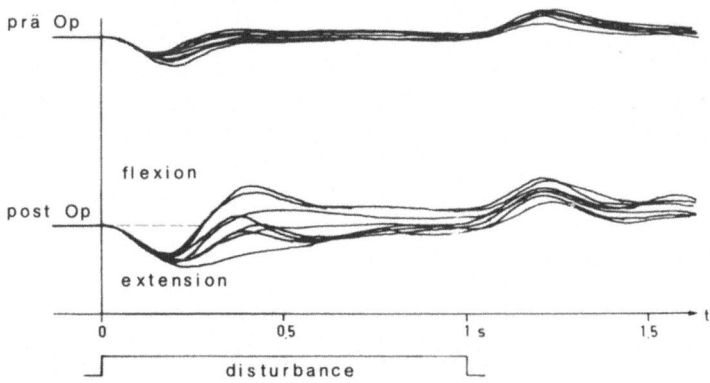

Fig. 2. Forearm position at "resist". Mechanographic recordings of stretch induced responses before (upper trace) and after operation (lower trace). The perturbation begins at 0 ms. The mechanical deviation of the forearm is recorded at the elbow joints. Note the larger mechanical deflection following operation.

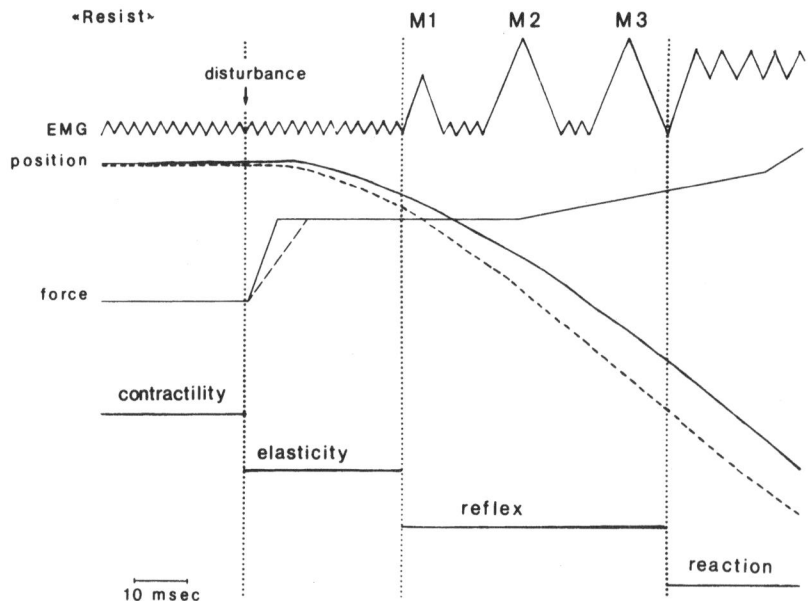

Fig. 3. Factors producing muscle stiffness during "resist". The dotted line represents the slope of a poststereotaxic patient (from Struppler, 1985).

Since we sometimes could observe that the elbow angular displacement following external perturbation appeared earlier on the hypotonic side in comparison to the normal side, even within the first 30 ms, the question arises: is this kind of hypotonia due to decreased reflex activity and additionally due to reduced non-reflex muscle stiffness?

The compensation of the external perturbation is an adaptive function of our motor system. Here we may theoretically discriminate 3 main functions:

1) contractility and elasticity of activated muscle, which counteract external disturbance;
2) proprioceptive reflexes, no matter whether spinally and/or supra-spinally mediated; and
3) voluntary compensation.

In order to investigate this problem, we try to quantify the muscle stiffness. With this methodology one can distinguish 2 modes of innervation serving muscle tone during isometric innervation:

1) early compensation of sudden external disturbances before reflex onset and
2) compensation via reflex arc.

In order to evaluate indirectly muscle stiffness, we have to measure the mechanogram and the dynamogram, using a force transducer placed between the lever of the machine and the arm of the patient.

Recording the dynamogram developed only by the torque motor under fixed conditions we will find a typical curve with well expressed local maxima and mechanical oscillations, superimposed on the curve. Analysing the time course of the human arm, however, local maximum shifts backward in the time and the oscillations are abolished.

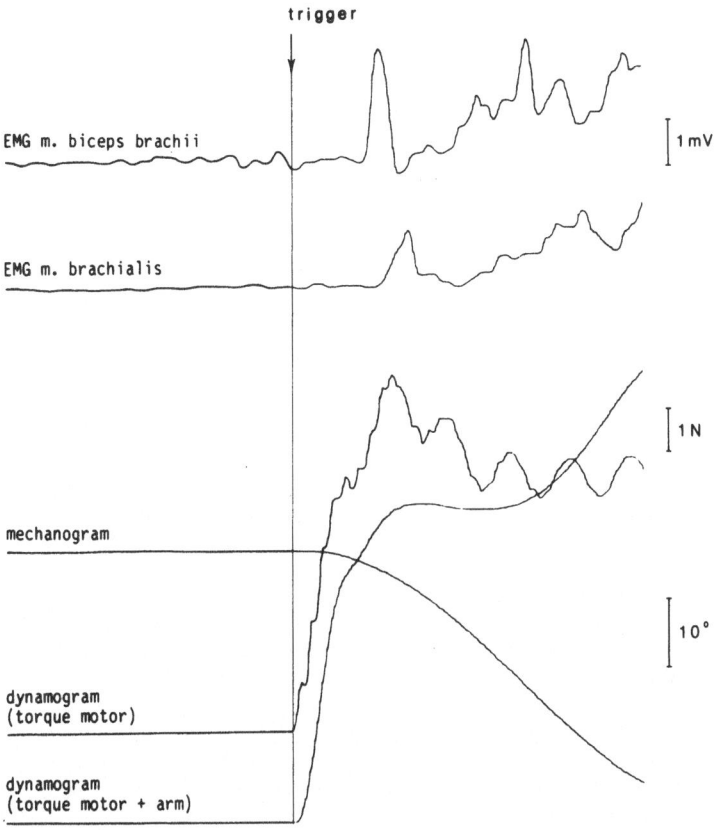

Fig. 4. Modification of mechanical parameters during torque disturbance.

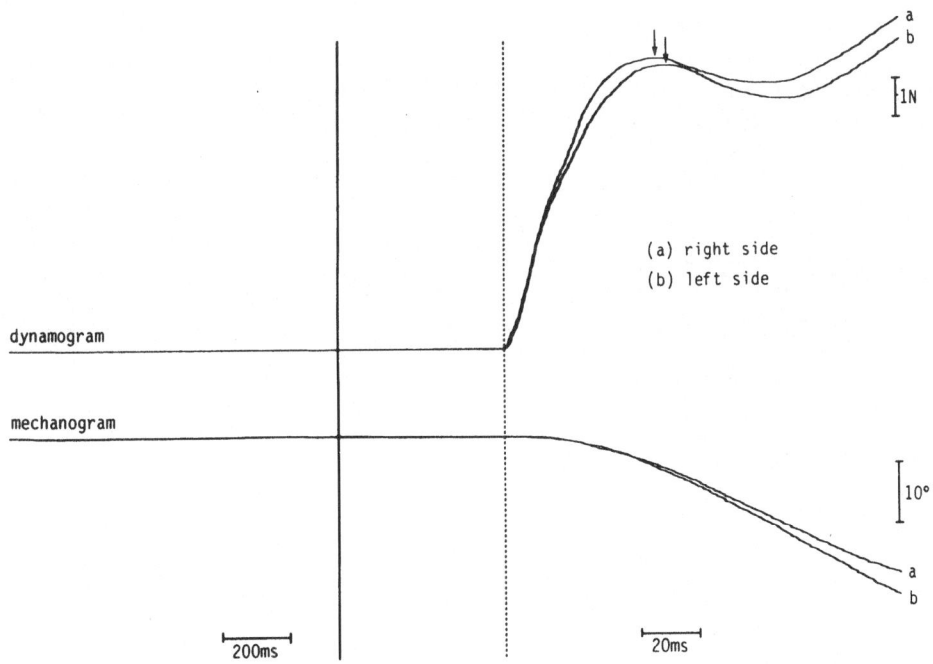

Fig. 5. Left side hypotonia following stereotaxic lesion. The latencies of the local maxima are longer at the hypotonic side.

We investigated patients showing slight contralateral 1-side-hypotonia following small stereotaxic lesions, measuring the latency of the local maxima and the dynamogram and the changes in the mechanogram.

The latencies of the local maxima are longer on the hypotonic side. The changes following perturbation are better expressed in the dynamogram than in the mechanogram. The absolute values of the latencies of the local maxima of both, operated and non-operated, side are shown in Figure 6.

How can we interpret these findings? Assuming the results of decreased muscle stiffness following stereotaxic lesions can further be confirmed, 2 mechanisms could be considered:

1) the original population of motor units generating the control movement is switched in a new one with different intrinsic mechanical properties and
2) the distribution of activity into the synergistic muscles is changed, in this case into the various forearm flexor muscles (brachialis, biceps and brachioradialis).

For immediate compensation of external perturbations muscle stiffness seems to be important. For this purpose we need probably a special feedback originating in the skeletal muscle for holding continuously the adequate ratio between muscle force and length.

If hypotonia of subthalamic-thalamic origin is more pronounced than that of peripheral origin like in polyneuropathies, one could assume a higher density in the representation of this afferent system at the thalamic level.

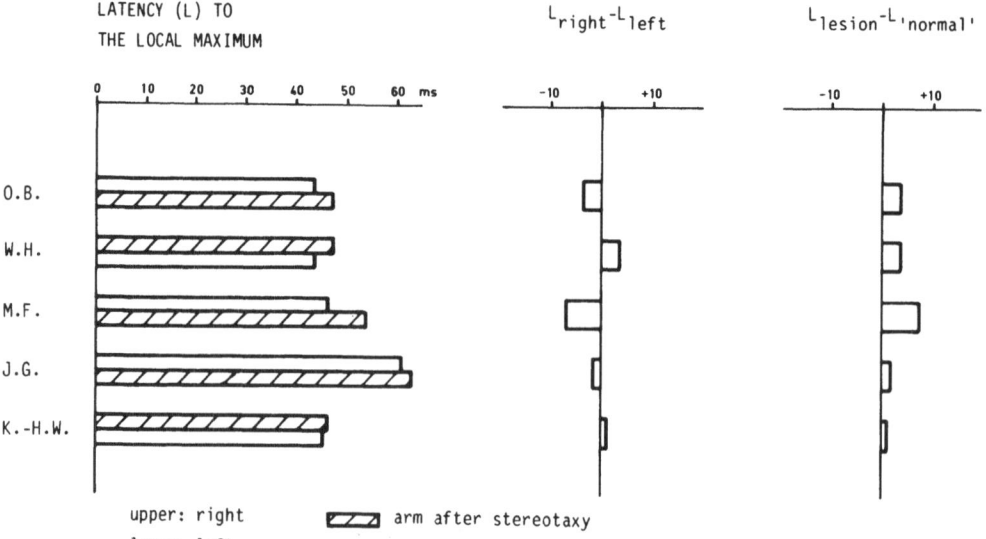

Fig. 6. Comparison of latencies between left (upper column) and right side (lower column) in 5 patients. The latency on the operated side (filled column) is longer.

SUMMARY

To differentiate whether hypotonia is due to decreased reflex activity and additionally reduced non-reflex muscle stiffness, torque-induced stretch responses in the forearm flexor muscles were investigated. In hypotonia following stereotaxic lesions on subthalamic-thalamic level the early compensation of sudden external disturbances is diminished <u>before</u> reflex onset. A special feedback system is discussed, originating in the skeletal muscle serving continuously the adequate muscle stiffness during sustained movements. This facilitatory system may have the highest density at thalamic level, in contrast to the representation in the peripheral nerve.

REFERENCES

Lehmann-Horn, F., Struppler, A., Klein, W., Lücking, C. H., Burgmayer, B., and Deuschl, G., 1982, Veränderungen der motorischen kontrolle bei Parkinson-patienten, <u>in</u>: "Elektrophysiologische Diagnostik in der Neurologie", A. Struppler, ed., pp. 236-237, G. Thieme Verlag, Stuttgart.

Struppler, A., 1985, Stereoencephalotomy and motor control, <u>in</u>: "Electro-myography and Evoked Potentials", A. Struppler and A. Weindl, eds., Springer-Verlag, Berlin, Heidelberg.

Tatton, W. G., and Lee, R. G., 1975, Motor responses to sudden upper limb displacements of the wrist in normal humans and parkinsonian patients, <u>Clin.Res.</u>, 22:755a.

PRESYNAPTIC INHIBITION AND DISINHIBITION

OF MONOSYNAPTIC REFLEX IN MAN

R. Person and G. Kozhina

Institute for Problems of Information Transmission
USSR Academy of Science
Moscow, USSR

The presynaptic inhibition is the object of intensive research mainly in acute animal experiments. But studies on intact human beings have the advantage of any neurophysiological mechanism. The presynaptic inhibition in the arc of monosynaptic reflex from spindles is accessible for such a study. Monosynaptic reflex can be modulated only by two ways: by change of motoneuron pool excitability and by presynaptic inhibition and disinhibition. The descending tonic presynaptic inhibition of soleus H-reflex in healthy man was shown by Delwaide (1973). Presynaptic inhibition in monosynaptic arc was revealed during rhythmic stimulation of Ia afferents (low-frequency depression) and during muscle vibration (see Rudomin, 1980).

One of the reliable ways to reveal the presynaptic inhibition effect in monosynaptic arc is to show the depression of the monosynaptic reflex during the activation of motoneurons via any other input. Our attention was drawn to the absence of H-reflex in some human muscles. It is impossible to evoke the H-reflex in hand muscles of most healthy people at rest and during contraction, but it appears in these muscles in persons with supraspinal lesion. This fact was known for a long time, especially to physicians, but its cause was not analysed.

The routine method of the H-reflex study has a certain limitation as the results of high strength stimulation are difficult to interpret because of a possibility of collision of orthodromic and antidromic volleys in motoneurons. We studied the effect of stimulation on single motor units (MUs). The muscle under study - abd.poll.br. or abd.dig.min. - was slightly voluntarily contracted and MU potentials were recorded. Against the background of this activity the corresponding nerve was repeatedly stimulated by single stimuli and peristimulus hystograms of single MUs were plotted. it is known that the smallest motoneurons have the lowest thresholds to the voluntary and reflex activation but their thin axons have the highest thresholds to electric stimulation. Therefore during weak contraction even a rather strong nerve stimulation does not activate the axon of firing MU. So the possibility of collision of ortho- and antidromic volleys in it is excluded.

Such experiments showed that the MUs of muscle under study did not respond monosynaptically either to weak or strong stimuli (Figure 1a,b). In the same muscles of subject suffering from CNS lesion a distinct response with latency of monosynaptic reflex (25 ms) was revealed

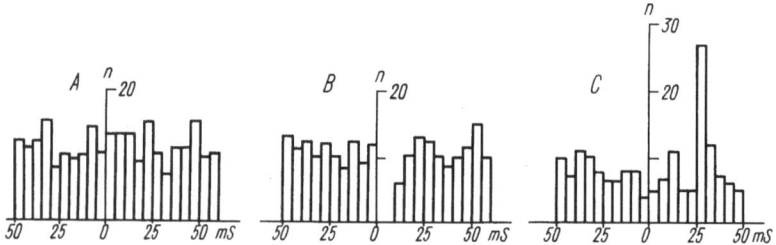

Fig. 1.   The effect of electric stimulation of hand muscle Ia afferents on
          the MU activity. Peristimulus histograms of single MUs. x-axis –
          time; y-axis – the number of MU potentials in the column; (A)
          healthy subject, weak stimuli; (B) the same, strong stimuli;
          M-response – 70% of M-max; (C) subject suffering from CNS lesion,
          weak stimuli.

(Figure 1c). Thus motoneuron pool of hand muscles of intact man did not
respond to activation of Ia afferents and at the same time did respond by
rhythmic firing to descending inflow. Therefore the inhibition of the
motoneuron itself cannot be a mechanism of the H-reflex suppression.
The alternative explanation of this suppression is the tonic presynaptic
inhibition apparently from the supraspinal levels of CNS.

In the above experiments the result of electric stimulation of Ia
afferents was studied. This nerve stimulation also activated part of
efferents (except those of firing MUs) and evoked the muscle twitch which
could be used to study the effect of the adequate influence on the
spindles. The monosynaptic effect of spindle unloading is usually regarded
as the main part of the silent period (SP) during the evoked twitch. As to
hand muscles this statement disagrees with the absence of the H-reflex in
these muscles. So we traced the events after the evoked twitch. The used
technique allowed to test the contribution of the monosynaptic effect from
spindles in the SP as an antidromic discharge in the motoneuron under study
did not occur and therefore the earliest component of the SP – the after-
hyperpolarization – was excluded.

In such experiments even during a rather strong twitch evoked by a
strong nerve stimulation the latency of the SP was no less than 60–70 ms as
measured from the stimulation and 50–60 ms as measured from the beginning
of muscle shortening (Figure 2a). It was too long for a monosynaptic
effect. So the first part of the SP during maximal twitch in these muscles
is the result of after-hyperpolarization of the motoneuron following its
antidromic discharge (Figure 2b). The long-latency SP could be the result
of the long-loop reflex from spindles (see below) and also the cutaneous
reflex as we saw from the SP with the same latency when the stimulating
electrode was shifted from the nerve so the stimulation did not evoke a
muscle twitch.

The most convincing way to reveal the effect of spindle shortening is
to study the unloading of muscle as in this case the muscle shortening
occurs without a stimulation, the background muscle activity is rather
strong and the velocity of shortening is very high. In such experiments
the SP latency was equal to 50 ms, i.e., was twice as much as the latency
of monosynaptic reflex (Figure 2c).

Thus in the investigated hand muscles of healthy man there is a
complete tonic presynaptic suppression of spinal monosynaptic reflex from
Ia afferents, both under their electric stimulation and during adequate

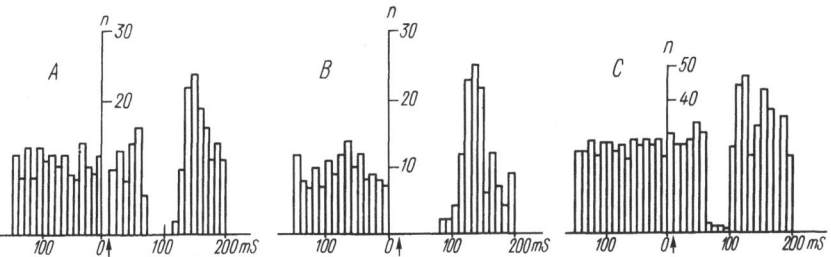

Fig. 2. The effect of hand muscle shortening on the MU activity. The
histograms as on Figure 1. The arrow – the beginning of muscle
shortening; (A) evoked twitch; M-response – 70% of M-max; (B)
maximal evoked twitch, the MUs under study were excited antidromically; (C) muscle unloading.

spindle disactivation, both at rest and during a rather high activity of
the muscle.

But there are some muscles such as tibial.ant. in which the H-reflex
is absent at rest but can be evoked during voluntary contraction. H-reflex
of soleus muscle is also facilitated during contraction. What is the
mechanism of such facilitation – the change of motoneuron pool state or
presynaptic disinhibition in the reflex arc?

Some authors compared the level of muscle activity during contraction
(using EMG) and the value of H-reflex. There was no correlation between
them and the increase of H-response took place mainly during the first part
of the contraction (Gottlieb et al., 1970; Pierrot-Deseilligny and Bussel,
1973). We traced the soleus H-reflex during a rather long-lasting contraction (5 s) with moderate strength (Figure 3). The constant level of
muscle contraction was verified by the EMG. Single and paired stimulation
was used (the interval in the pair was equal to 0.5 s). Under such paired
stimulation at rest the first stimulus activated the presynaptic inhibition
in monosynaptic arc and the second H-response was decreased (low-frequency
depression). At the beginning of the contraction the amplitude of response
to stimuli increased significantly but during 500 to 600 ms the H-response
considerably decreased and its value became settled on a rather constant
level slightly higher than the value at rest. We consider the absence of
correlation between the value of H-reflex facilitation and the level of
motoneuron pool activity to be the result of the interference of the presynaptic disinhibition which, apparently, accompanies only the early part
of voluntary muscle contraction. The weak constant H-reflex facilitation
during the rest of the long contraction may be due to the activated state
of motoneuron pool, mainly owing to the existence of underthreshold fringe.
The experiments also showed that the presynaptic inhibition under paired
stimulation disappeared completely all along muscle contraction.

Some conclusions can be drawn from the above data. Complete presynaptic suppression of monosynaptic reflex from spindles in hand muscles,
both at rest and in contraction state shows that this reflex is not
necessary for muscle contraction control. The complete suppression may be
due to the high corticalization of muscle control. Apparently, the presynaptic inhibition controls the H-reflex in other muscles even in soleus
in which this reflex is higher than in any other muscle but, nevertheless,
is tonically suppressed to some extent. During the beginning of the voluntary muscle contraction a presynaptic disinhibition of monosynaptic arc
takes place. Besides, the voluntary contraction abolishes low-frequency
depression, i.e., the negative feedback in the monosynaptic arc itself.

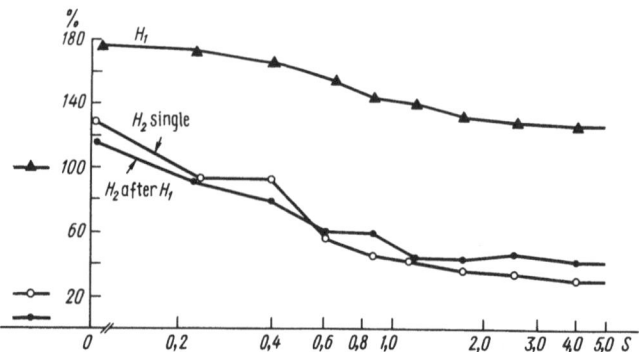

Fig. 3. The H-reflex of soleus during steady voluntary contraction (3
experiments). x-axis - time; y-axis - the amplitude of H-reflex,
% of H-max. Single and paired stimulation by strong (H_1) and weak
(H_2) stimuli. On the left - the amplitudes of H-reflex at rest.

Rack (1981) gives careful consideration to the problem of the role of
somatosensory feedback in motor control. He argues that the gain of the
stretch reflex has to be low to avoid the uncontrollable oscillations in
motor system due to long conducting delay. But under some circumstances
reflex feedback control of motor activity is used. It is possible as the
gain of the reflex may be modulated. According to this point of view the
H-reflex suppression and the H-reflex changes during long-lasting muscle
contraction in our experiments may get a functional explanation.

REFERENCES

Delwaide, P. J., 1973, Human monosynaptic reflexes and presynaptic inhi-
        bition, in: "New Developments in Electromyography and Clinical
        Neurophysiology", J. E. Desmedt, ed., vol. 3, Karger, Basel.
Gottlieb, G. L., Agarval, G. C., and Stark, L., 1970, Interaction between
        voluntary and postural mechanisms of the human motor system, J.
        Neurophysiol., 33:365.
Pierrot-Deseilligny, E., and Bussel, B., 1973, A comparison of H-reflex at
        the onset of a voluntary movement or a polysynaptic reflex, Brain
        Res., 60:482.
Rack, P. M. N., 1981, Limitation of somatosensory feedback in control of
        posture and movement, in: "Handbook of Physiology," Section 1, Vol.
        2, V. B. Brooks, ed., Amer. Physiol. Soc., Bethesda.
Rudomin, P., 1980, Information processing at synapses in the vertebrate
        spinal cord: presynaptic control of information transfer in mono-
        synaptic pathways, in: "Information Processing in the Nervous
        System", H. Pinsker, ed., Raven Press, New York.

THE DIFFERENTIATION OF GOLGI TENDON ORGANS IN THE RAT

HIND LIMB MUSCLES AFTER NEONATAL DE-EFFERENTATION

T. Soukup and J. Zelená

Institute of Physiology
Czechoslovak Academy of Sciences
Prague, Czechoslovakia

SUMMARY

After neonatal de-efferentation, the size of tendon organs (TOs) in the rat changes due to the resulting immobilization of the hind limbs. The mean length of TOs increases and the width decreases in extensor digitorum longus muscles which become stretched, whereas opposite changes occur in soleus muscles which become shortened after de-efferentation. The differentiation of the fine structural features of TOs is, however, unimpaired by de-efferentation. It thus can be concluded that elimination of muscle contraction and tension does not prevent the differentiation of basic structural properties of TOs deprived of adequate stimulation during their postnatal morphogenesis.

INTRODUCTION

The development of mammalian stretch receptors is triggered and maintained by their innervation (Zelená, 1964; 1975). In the rat, the differentiation of stretch receptors is arrested after neonatal denervation and skeletal muscles remain devoid of muscle spindles and tendon organs even when they become reinnervated (Zelená and Hník, 1963). It was of interest to learn whether or not the differentiation of TOs would be impaired by permanent loss of muscle function and elimination of functional load of these mechanoreceptors following de-efferentation of skeletal muscles at birth. A part of these results has been published (Soukup and Zelená, 1985).

MATERIALS AND METHODS

The de-efferentation was performed in newborn Wistar rats by the extirpation of the lumbosacral spinal cord (Zelená and Soukup, 1974; 1985). This operation resulted in irreversible destruction of the motor innervation of the hind limbs, whereas spinal ganglia and sensory innervation were left intact. Extensor digitorum longus (EDL) and soleus (SOL) muscles of 3 to 16 week-old control and operated rats were either stained for cholinesterase (ChE) activity in toto (Silver, 1963) or processed for electron miscroscopy as described earlier (Soukup and Zelená, 1985). After staining for ChE, TOs were isolated and measured under a binocular microscope with an ocular miscrometer (Soukup, 1983).

Changes in Size of Tendon Organs after De-efferentation

Under normal conditions, the TOs from EDL and SOL muscles do not differ in their mean length and width, although considerable difference in size can exist between individual TOs in both muscles (Soukup, 1983). In 3 week-old rats, the mean length of TOs in the EDL and SOL muscles was 218 ± 8 µm (± S.E.) and 210 ± 6 µm, and the mean width 50 ± 2 µm and 49 ± 2 µm, respectively (Soukup and Zelená, 1985). Three weeks after neonatal de-efferentation, however, the TOs became on the average significantly longer and thinner in EDL muscles which were lengthened due to immobilization, whereas opposite alteration in the mean length and width of TOs occurred in SOL muscles which became shortened (Figure 1). The difference in the mean length (EDL: 255 ± 13 µm, SOL: 166 ± 5 µm) and width (EDL: 36 ± 1 µm, SOL: 55 ± 2 µm) of TOs in the two de-efferented muscles studied thus became highly significant (p<0.01). The differences in size between individual TOs in the same muscle remained, however, considerable after de-efferentation (Soukup and Zelená, 1985).

Ultrastructure of Tendon Organ after De-efferentation

The ultrastructural differentiation of TOs proceeded in de-efferented muscles as under normal conditions, and no significant abnormality was found in the fine structure of TOs examined 3-16 weeks after the operation. The capsule, the receptor body with collagen bundles and the sensory Ib fiber with its terminals (Figure 2) exhibited the same characteristics as in control tendon organs. Both the neurotendinous and purely collagenous compartments were formed as under normal conditions (cf. Zelená and Soukup, 1983; Soukup and Zelená, 1985).

Occurrence of Unmyelinated Axons in Tendon Organs

In normal TOs the Ib fiber is, as a rule, accompanied by several unmyelinated axons (Zelená and Soukup, 1983). This accessory innervation was also found in the TOs after de-efferentation. Several unmyelinated

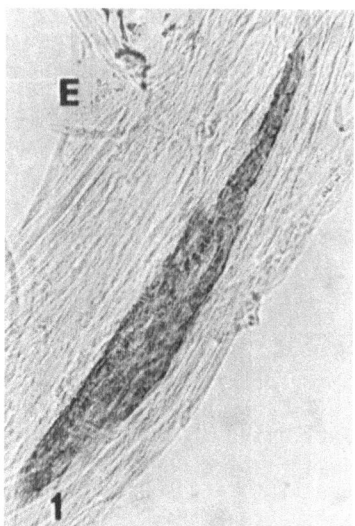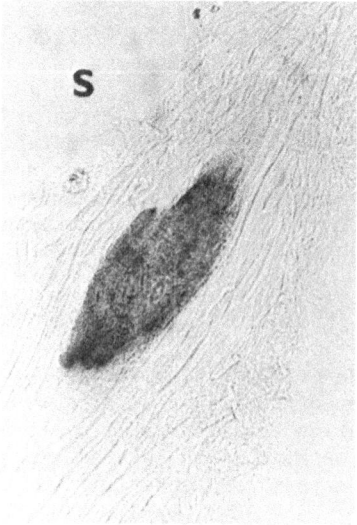

Fig. 1. Tendon organs stained for cholinesterase activity, from a 3-week-old rat de-efferented at birth. (E) an elongated and thin TO from an EDL muscle; (S) a short and wide TO from a SOL muscle. x210.

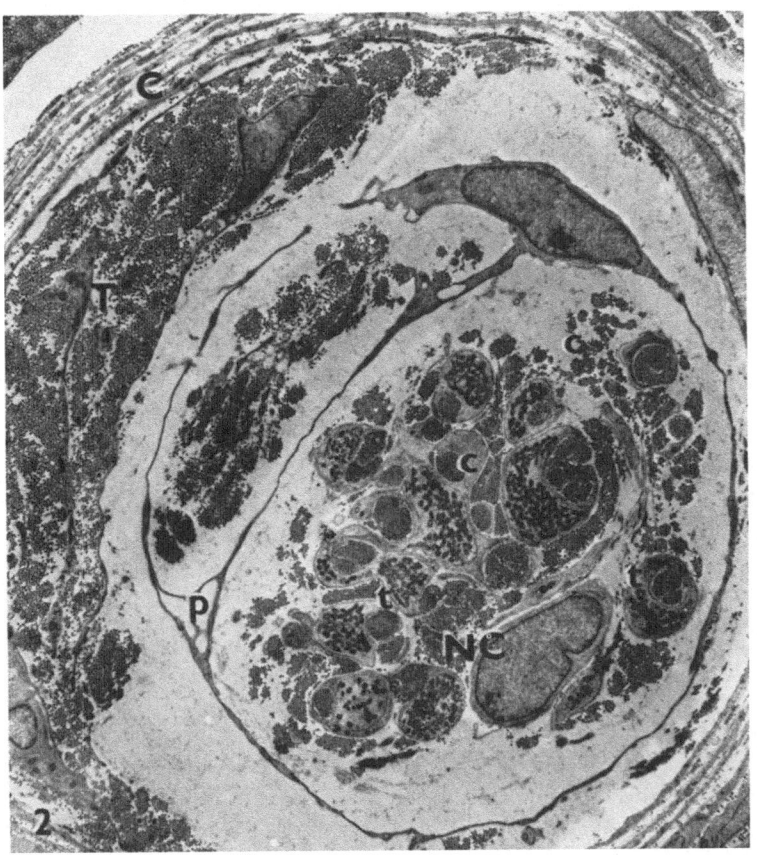

Fig. 2. Transverse section of a tendon organ from de-efferented soleus
muscle of a 7-week-old rat. Neurotendinous compartment (NC)
contains complex axon terminals (t) and discrete collagen bundles
(c); it is separated by septal partitions (p) and fluid-filled
spaces from tendinous compartment (T) composed of densely packed
collagen bundles; (C) capsule. x5000.

axons in one or two groups coursed along with the Ib fiber up to the TO.
A part of them, however, left the common perineurial sheath outside the
TO and joined the blood vessels in the vicinity of the capsule. Other
unmyelinated axons entered the capsule and ran between the capsular
lamellae near the capillaries (Figure 3) or a part of them. Occasionally,
1-3 unmyelinated axons followed the Ib branches in their intracapsular
course and could be found in the lumen of the TO.

CONCLUSIONS

     In contrast to the deleterious effect of denervation (Zelená and Hník,
1963), de-efferentation of skeletal muscles does not significantly affect
the development and ultrastructural differentiation of TOs. After the
latter operation, TOs differentiated with normal ultrastructural features,
but their growth and mean size become changed in accord with the changes in
length of the disused muscles. It can be concluded that elimination of
muscle function during the period of postnatal development indirectly
affects the mean size of TOs, but does not otherwise interfere with their
morphogenesis.

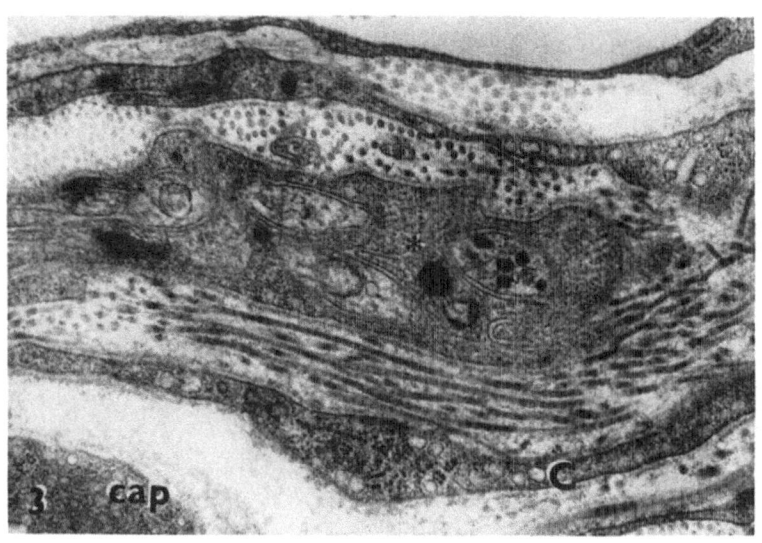

Fig. 3. A group of unmyelinated nerve fibers (asterisk) 0.1-0.3 μm in
diameter, localized within a common Schwann cell among the laminae
of the capsule (C) of a TO near an intracapsular capillary (cap).
De-efferented SOL muscle of a 7-week-old rat. x30000.

As regards the innervation of TOs by unmyelinated axons, their
character and functional significance remain to be elucidated in further
experiments.

REFERENCES

Silver, A., 1963, A histochemical investigation of cholinesterases at
neuromuscular junctions in mammalian and avian muscle, J.Physiol.,
169:386.
Soukup, T., 1983, The number, distribution and size of Golgi tendon organs
in the developing and adult rat muscles, Physiol.Bohemoslov.,
32:211.
Soukup, T., and Zelená, J., 1985, Structure of tendon organs of the rat
after de-efferentation, Cell Tiss.Res., 241:229.
Zelená, J., 1964, Development, degeneration and regeneration of receptor
organs, Progr.Brain Res., 13:175.
Zelená, J., 1975, The role of sensory innervation in the development of
mechanoreceptors, Progr.Brain Res., 43:49.
Zelená, J., and Hník, P., 1967, Effect of innervation on the development of
muscle receptors, in: "The Effect of Use and Disuse on Neuromuscular
Functions", E. Gutmann and P. Hník, eds., p. 95, Academia, Prague.
Zelená, J., and Soukup, T., 1974, The differentiation of intrafusal fiber
types in rat muscle spindles after motor denervation, Cell Tiss.
Res., 153:115.
Zelená, J., and Soukup, T., 1983, The in-series and in-parallel components
of rat tendon organs, Neuroscience, 9:899.

SECTION III
CENTRAL CONTROL OF MOVEMENTS

TRIGEMINAL AFFERENTS TO THE FASTIGIAL N. AND PALEOCEREBELLAR MODULATION OF
HYPOGLOSSAL MOTONEURONS: NEUROANATOMICAL AND ELECTROPHYSIOLOGICAL STUDY
SUGGESTING A TRANSCEREBELLAR LOOP FOR TONGUE MUSCLE ACTIVITY REGULATION

A. Bava, F. Fabbro, S. Mininel-Conte, G. Leanza*
A. Russo*, and S. Stanzani*
Institutes of Physiology
University of Trieste and
*Catania, Italy

Cerebellar control and trigeminal afferents appear to have both,
individually or in coordination, determining roles in the regulation of
motor activities such as suction, mastication, vocalization and speech
(see Luschei and Goldberg, 1981; Grillner et al., 1982). Assuming the
functional importance for such motor activities of close relationships
between trigeminal afferents, paleocerebellum and trigeminal, facial and
hypoglossal efferents, we began a series of experiments, using both electrophysiological and neuroanatomical methods.

The first study referred in this paper, as an extension of the results
obtained during previous work (see Bava et al., 1972), was undertaken with
the intent to ascertain the nature and the functional properties of the
paleocerebellar nuclear influences on single hypoglossal (XII) motoneurons,
to further elucidate some characteristics of the cerebellar control of the
tongue motility (see Bowman and Aldes, 1980).

The experiments were performed on 10 rabbits, anesthetized with chlor-
alose-nembutal admixture (50-30 mg/kg i.p.), or in some cases decerebrated
at midcollicular level. The animals were curarized and artificially ven-
tilated (alveolar pCO_2 being continuously monitored). The lingual and XII
nerves were dissected out for subsequent stimulation. Bipolar concentric
electrodes (0.5 mm in outer diameter; 50 µm at the tip; impedance 200 KΩ)
were inserted under stereotaxic guidance into the fastigial nucleus contralateral to the hypoglossal nucleus chosen for recording. Fastigial stimuli
were square waves of 0.1-0.5 msec duration and 2.5-7.5 V amplitude,
delivered alone or in short trains of 3-6 pulses at 100-320/sec. Spontaneous or evoked activity of hypoglossal motoneurons was intra- and/or juxta-
cellularly recorded by glass capillary micropipettes filled with a 2.0 M
K-citrate solution (tip diameter less than 0.5 µm; 5-40 MΩ). The effects
evoked by paleocerebellar nuclear stimulation were tested: a) on the motoneurons spontaneous discharge; and b) on the unitary activity evoked by
trigeminal afferents [physiological (mechanical, and proprioceptive)
stimuli or electrical stimulation of lingual nerve], by intranuclear activation of hypoglossal nucleus, and by antidromic hypoglossal nerve stimulation. Motoneurons within the XII nucleus were identified by their antidromic response to low-intensity stimulation (0.1 to 5.0 mA, 0.1 msec) of
the XII nerve. The antidromic response was identified as a consistent,
"all-or-none" response with a short latency (less than 3.0 msec) to stimulation rates of 100 to 200/sec. All the neurons of our sample were anti-

dromically reactive to the XII nerve stimulation (see Lowe, 1978). After every experiment, the locations of both recording and stimulating electrodes were checked histologically on serial sections with the usual techniques of track reconstruction and/or electrolytic marking.

The experimental results were obtained from over 50 hypoglossal motoneurons; in 23 of them, the tape-recorded activities were fully processed off-line by computer analysis (poststimulus-time histograms, PSTHs). Contralateral fastigial nucleus stimulation was tested in all the hypoglossal motoneurons of our sample, being effective in 78% of the population. Different response patterns were evoked by the paleocerebellar nuclear stimulation: primary hyperpolarization (200-1500 msec in duration), pure (38%) or followed by postinhibitory rebound (30%), and, less frequently, pure excitation (10%); 22% of the analyzed hypoglossal motoneurons were unreactive to the cerebellar stimulation.

Different response patterns (inhibitory and excitatory effects) could sometimes be evoked, by contralateral fastigial nucleus stimulation, on the spontaneous activity of the same hypoglossal motoneuron, depending on the duration of the paleocerebellar nuclear stimulation (see data in Bava, 1985). Therefore the possibility exists that impulses of paleocerebellar origin can modulate the reactivity of motoneuron activities related to the neural regulation of tongue movements. It is well known that the vermal cortex of the anterior lobe and the fastigial nucleus of the cerebellum can control the activity of spinal motoneurons; the cerebellar stimulation evokes both inhibitory and excitatory effects (see data in Terzuolo, 1959 and Ito, 1984). Inhibitory effects were also exerted by the paleocerebellar nuclear stimulation on the hypoglossal motoneurons' activity evoked transsynaptically (see Figure 1, A-A'). The duration of the fastigial evoked inhibitory effect, which ranged from 200 to 1500 msec, was always directly related to the durations of paleocerebellar nuclear stimulation. Sometimes the fastigial nucleus stimulation produces facilitatory effects on the transsynaptic activities evoked in hypoglossal motoneurons (see Figure 1, B-B'). The inhibitory effect (200-1500 msec in duration) evoked by the paleocerebellar stimulation was also effective on antidromically induced firing in hypoglossal motoneurons. A spike potential evoked by antidromic stimulation is usually difficult to block by means of cerebellar inhibition (Terzuolo, 1959). In many instances, only the inflection present on the rising phase of the spike becomes more prominent (see Figure 2, A'); seldom, a partial block becomes evident (see Figure 2, B'). However, when two spikes are initiated within short time interval, the second one can always be partially (or completely) blocked as a result of cerebellar inhibition (see Figure 2, A'-B'). The blockade occurs between the IS and SD spike (Eccles, 1957).

Following the same line of research, in a subsequent study, we tried to define the projections from the brainstem trigeminal complex (sensory nucleus of the trigeminal nerve, NST, and nucleus of the spinal tract of the trigeminal nerve, NTST; Pellegrino et al., 1979) to the cerebellar fastigial nucleus, in adult rats, by using neuroanatomical methods, stereotaxic techniques, and retrograde labeling procedure utilizing a fluorescent substance ("Fast Blue", F.B.).

Experiments were performed on 20 male Wistar rats weighing 250-300 gm. The animals were anesthetized with alcohol (12.5% i.p.), and F.B. (4% in distilled water) was injected in the boundaries of the fastigial nucleus between stereotaxic planes -9.4/-10.4 (according to Pellegrino et al., 1979; see Figure 3, A). Injections were made by the aid of Hamilton microsyringe installed on a stereotaxic apparatus. After a survival time of 40 hours, the animals were anesthetized once again (alcohol 12.5% i.p.), sacrificed and perfused intracardially with saline solution, followed by

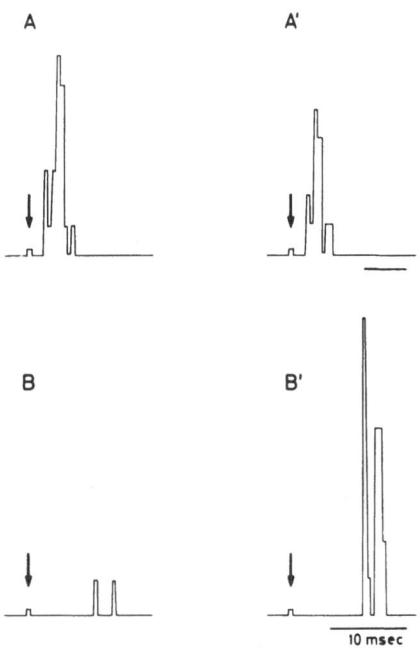

Fig. 1.   Effects of fastigial stimulation on unitary transsynaptic
          potentials evoked in the hypoglossal nucleus. (A-A') PSTHs
          (50 trials) obtained from the responses of a single hypoglossal
          motoneuron transsynaptically excited by intranuclear stimulation
          (arrows point out the stimulation artefacts). In (A') inhibitory
          effect evoked on the computed unitary activity by paleocerebellar
          stimulation (prior activation of the contralateral fastigial
          nucleus: 35 msec; three shocks at 320/sec). (B-B') PSTHs
          (50 trials) obtained from the unitary responses of a different
          hypoglossal motoneuron transsynaptically excited by stimulation of
          the lingual nerve (arrows point out the stimulation artefacts).
          In (B') facilitatory effect evoked on the computed unitary
          activity by paleocerebellar stimulation (prior activation of the
          contralateral fastigial nucleus: 50 msec; three shocks at
          320/sec).

buffered phosphate 15% formaline (pH 7.4). The brains were removed and
immediately transferred to a freezing microtome. Frozen coronal sections
of the brains were obtained at a thickness of 40 μm. The sections were
then examined with a Polyvar Reichert fluorescence microscope and photo-
graphed with an automatic camera.

        After accurate F.B. microinjections (0.04 μl) in the fastigial nucleus
of one side labeled neurons were found only in the NTST, both ipsilateral
and contralateral to the injected side. As it is known (see Hayashi et
al., 1984) three cytoarchitectonically different subnuclei compose the
NTST: subnucleus oralis, interpolaris, and caudalis. Carefully considering
the anatomical boundaries of the three NTST subdivisions, the F.B.-labeled
trigemino-fastigial neurons were found to have a distribution restricted to
the subnucleus interpolaris and to the rostral section of the subnucleus
caudalis of both sides (stereotaxic planes -9.0/-13.4). Particularly, a
prevalent localization of the F.B.-labeled trigemino-fastigial neurons was
constantly found between the stereotaxic planes -11/-13.0 (see Figure 3,
B), and in the ventrolateral regions of the subnuclei interpolaris and
caudalis. In the NTST contralateral to the injected fastigial nucleus the

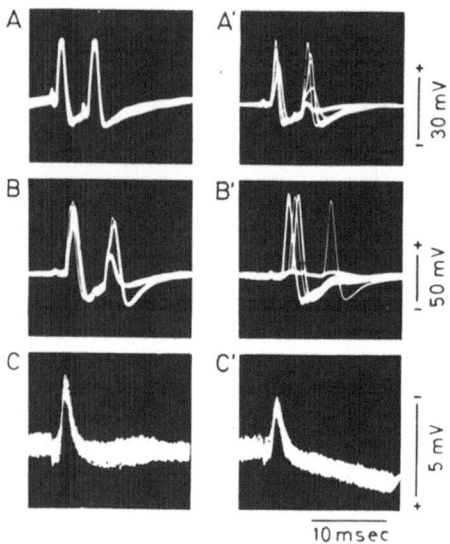

Fig. 2. Effects of fastigial stimulation on unitary and focal antidromic
potentials evoked in the hypoglossal nucleus (activation of the
central end of the homonymous XII nerve). (A) intracellular
recording (superimposed sweeps) from a hypoglossal motoneuron
showing a series of evoked antidromic responses (double shocks at
250/sec). (A') as a result of paleocerebellar nuclear stimulation
(prior activation of the contralateral fastigial nucleus: 50 msec;
three shocks at 320/sec), partial or total block of the portion of
the spikes which follow the initial one it obtained. The blockade, as a result of cerebellar inhibition, occurs between the IS
and SD spike (Eccles, 1957). (B) intracellular recording (superimposed sweeps) from a different hypoglossal motoneuron, showing a
series of evoked antidromic responses (double shocks at 200/sec;
note, in this case, the blockade that occurs in the second unitary
response between the IS and SD spike). (B') as a result of paleocerebellar nuclear stimulation (performed as in (A')), partial or
total block of the evoked antidromic responses again occurs, as a
result of the cerebellar inhibition. (C-C') different preparation. In (C') the inhibitory effect evoked by the paleocerebellar stimulation (performed as in (A')) on the focal antidromic
potential elicited in the hypoglossal nucleus is also evident.

F.B.-labeled neurons were always less numerous and with a less intense blue
fluorescent cytoplasm, as compared to the F.B.-labeled neurons in the
homonymous regions of the ipsilateral NTST (see Figure 3, B). The F.B.-
labeled, trigemino-fastigial, NTST neurons were found to have multipolar
and fusiform cell bodies, of large (40 μm), medium (20 μm) and small
(10 μm) size.

    In agreement with our experimental results and according to our hy-
pothesis, the consistency of the NTST bilateral projections on to the
paleocerebellar nuclear structures and the functional characteristics of
the effects exerted by the fastigial nucleus efferents on to the hypoglossal motoneurons, through the complex nature of the trigeminal sensory
information, could contribute to the cerebellar control exerted on the
tongue motor functions in connection with the oral and perioral integrated
processes, swiftly, without involving the intricate cerebellar cortical
machinery.

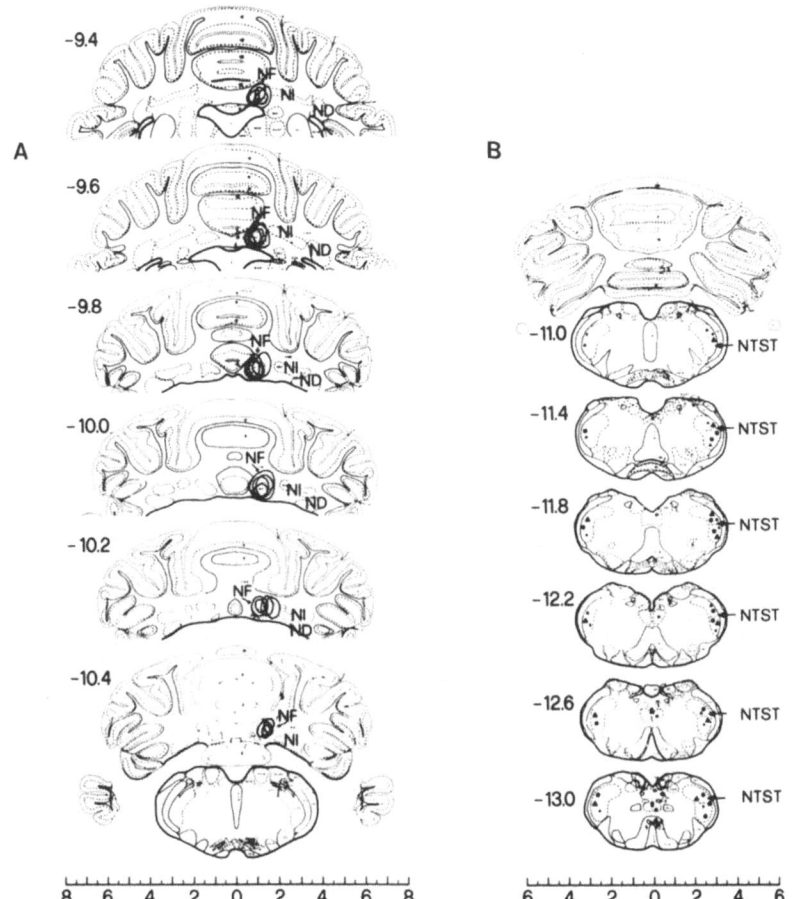

Fig. 3.   The figure shows, in (A), in successive coronal sections of the
rat cerebellum, the extension of the "Fast Blue" (F.B.) injections
in, and around, the boundaries of the fastigial nucleus (NF) of
the right side, between the stereotaxic planes -9.4/-10.4 (see
Pellegrino et al., 1979). NI: interpositus nucleus; ND: dentate
nucleus.   The figure also shows, in (B), in successive coronal
sections, the localization of F.B.-labeled trigemino-fastigial
neurons in the nucleus of the spinal tract of the trigeminal nerve
(NTST), subnucleus interpolaris (stereotaxic planes -11.0/-12.2;
see Pellegrino et al., 1979), and subnucleus caudalis (stereotaxic
planes -12.6/13.0), following a single F.B. injection in the NF of
the right side.   In the ipsilateral side of injection the labeled
NTST neurons are more numerous, than in the contralateral one.
Note the intranuclear distribution of the trigemino-fastigial
neurons.   The large and small triangles indicate large and small
multipolar cells, respectively; the large and small circles indicate large and small fusiform cells, respectively.   Scales in mm.

REFERENCES

Bava, A., 1985, Fisiologia del sistema nervoso, in: "Trattato di Foniatria
    e Logopedia," Vol. I, Anatomia e Fisiologia degli organi della
    comunicazione, pp.167-222, L. Croatto, ed., Editrice 'La Garangola,'
    Padova.

Bava, A., Innocenti, G. M., and Raffaele, R., 1972, Effects exerted by trigeminal and fastigial stimulation on Staderini's nucleus intercalatus, Arch.Sci.biol., 56:13-34.

Bowman, J. P. and Aldes, L. D., 1980, Organization of the cerebellar tongue representation in the monkey, Exp.Brain Res., 39:249-259.

Eccles, J. C., 1957, "The Physiology of Nerve Cells," The Johns Hopkins Press, Baltimore, MD.

Grillner, S., Lindblom, B., Lubker, J., Persson, A., eds., 1982, "Speech Motor Control,"; Proc. Int. Symp. on Speech Motor Control, Wenner-Gren Center, Stockholm, May 11 and 12, 1981, Pergamon Press; Oxford, New York and Toronto.

Hayashi, H., Sumino, R., and Sessle, B. J., 1984, Functional organization of trigeminal subnucleus interpolaris: nociceptive and innocuous afferent inputs, projections to thalamus, cerebellum, and spinal cord, and descending modulation from periaqueductal gray, J.Neurophysiol., 51:890-905.

Ito, M., 1984, "The Cerebellum and Neural Control," Raven Press, New York.

Lowe, A. A., 1978, Excitatory and inhibitory inputs to hypoglossal motoneurons and adjacent reticular formation neurons in cats, Exp.Neurol., 62:30-47.

Luschei, E. S. and Goldberg, L. J., 1981, Neural mechanisms of mandibular control: mastication and voluntary biting, in: "Handbook of Physiology," Sect. 1, The Nervous System; Vol. II, Motor Control, Part 2, pp.1237-1274, J. M. Brookhart, V. B. Brooks, S. R. Geiger, V. B. Mountcastle, eds., Amer. Physiol. Soc., Bethesda, MD.

Pellegrino, L. J., Pellegrino, A. S., and Cushman, A. J., 1979, "A Stereotaxic Atlas of the Rat Brain," Plenum Press, New York and London.

Terzuolo, C. A., 1959, Cerebellar inhibitory and excitatory actions upon spinal extensor motoneurons, Arch.Ital.Biol., 97:316-339.

EMG AND HIPPOCAMPAL EEG ACTIVITIES DURING SPONTANEOUS

AND ELICITED MOVEMENTS IN THE RAT

R. Korczyński, S. Kasicki, and U. Borecka*

Department of Neurophysiology, Nencki Institute of
Experimental Biology, and *Department of Bionics,
Institute of Biocybernetics and Biomedical Engineering
Warsaw

INTRODUCTION

The relationship between the hippocampal rhythmical slow activity
(RSA) and the process of execution of movement, observed by a number of
authors may suggest involvement of hippocampal formation in higher level
control of the motor processes (Whishaw and Vanderwolf 1973). The main
conclusion is that higher-frequency RSA (7-12 Hz) accompanies 'volitional'
movements (e.g., locomotion, lever pressing) as opposed to 'automatic'
movements (e.g., scratching, drinking) when lower-frequency of RSA (4-7 Hz)
or desynchronization occurs. The amplitude of RSA during the 'volitional'
movement has been found to be related to the number of muscles engaged
while the frequency of RSA reflects the rate of acceleration.

The aim of the present study was to examine the frequency of hippocampal RSA under different experimental conditions during locomotion or
other locomotor-like behaviors.

MATERIAL AND METHODS

The detailed description is to be published elsewhere (Korczyński and
Kasicki 1986, Korczyński 1986). Briefly: hippocampal EEG and limb EMG were
chronically recorded in twenty-one male rats. Copper-nickel wires enameled
with polyurethane (ϕ = 193 μm, The Sci. Wire Co. London) were bilaterally
implanted into the dorsal hippocampus whereas EMG bipolar, nichrome wires
(ϕ = 100 μm) were implanted into the following muscles: tibialis anterior,
soleus and/or triceps and biceps. The recorded potentials were filtered at
4-7 Hz and 8-13 Hz bands, and fed into an ink-writing polygraph and an
oscilloscope.

The apparatus consisted of home cage and a runway alley. The home
cage was an inverted, truncated pyramid with a base of 22 x 40 cm and
height of 18 cm. It was equipped with a sawdust cushioned floor and opened
at the top. The runway alley, 160 cm long and 10 cm wide, had a 'start-
platform' (a plate of 17 × 17 cm) at one end and a 'goal box' (a wooden
cubic cage of 35 cm in length with the opened front) at the other. All
experiments were carried out in a weakly illuminated room with an electric
bulb positioned over the start platform.

The following tests were used:

(1) for quadrupedal locomotion a) spontaneous or tail pinch-induced locomotion in the home cage, b) the runway alley locomotion with the
animal trained to escape from the start platform to the goal box,
where it was allowed to rest for minimum 10 min.
(2) for locomotion on the forelimbs with the experimentor holding the
animals tail (the hindlimbs were not allowed to touch the runway
surface), either in the home cage or runway alley.
(3) for spontaneous movements on the animal lifted by the tail above the
home cage.
(4) for passive movements evoked by consecutive alternative pressure (with
two pencils) on the plantar region in the hindlimbs of the animal
being held vertically erect.

All tests were performed alternatively at random for three months,
with daily sessions up to two hours.

RESULTS

Quadrupedal locomotion tested in home cage, when spontaneous or
induced by a weak tail pinch, was always accompanied by RSA of 8 Hz or
more. However, during the early stages of instrumental conditioning in the
new environment of runway alley some rats performed locomotor movements
with RSA frequency of 7 Hz, which shifted during consecutive sessions to
the typical frequency of above 8 Hz (see Figure 1).

Lifting of the caudal part of the animal by holding its tail could
cause bipedal locomotion on the forelimbs, which was not accompanied by
rhythmical movements of hindlimbs, or any EMG rhythm in hindlimb, tested
muscles (see Figure 2). However, RSA accompanying this bipedal locomotion
had a frequency 7 Hz in some rats although in others the frequency rose
above 8 Hz. With consecutive training in all rats lower frequencies of RSA
changed to 8 Hz or more. It is interesting that such an increase in RSA
frequency tended to occur earlier in the runway alley than in home cage.

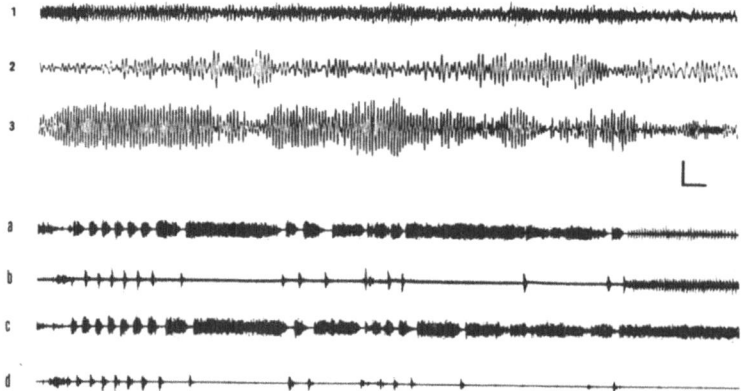

Fig. 1.   Hippocampal RSA and hindlimbs EMG activity during quadrupedal
          locomotion in the runway alley ended with scratching. (1) raw
          EEG; (2,3) bandpass filtered 4-7 Hz and 8-13 Hz respectively;
          (a,b) EMG of soleus and tibialis anterior left and (c,d) right
          respectively. Calibrations: horizontal 1 sec, vertical 200 μV
          and 1 mV. Note desynchronization during scratching.

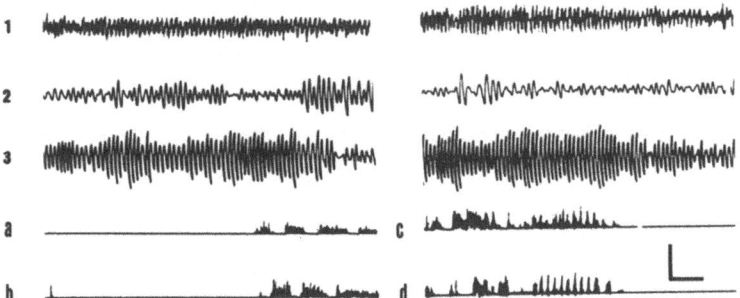

Fig. 2. Hippocampal RSA and fore- and hindlimbs integrated EMG activity
during bipedal locomotion in the runway alley in two rats A and B.
(1) raw EEG; (2,3) bandpass filtered 4-7 Hz and 8-13 Hz respectively; (a,b) EMG of soleus left and right and (c,d) lateral head
of triceps left and right. Calibrations as in Figure 1.

Lifting of the animal by the tail could result in initial immobilization which was soon followed by rhythmical alternative movements of
forelimbs, whereas the hindlimbs did not move. Prolonged lifting resulted
in vigorous rotations and/or flexions of the body, and other symptoms of
strong behavioral excitation. During such behavior the RSA frequency was
not stable and consisted of short-lasting episodes of large amplitude
irregular EEG or RSA of 7 Hz. Under such conditions the typical 8 Hz RSA
was not observed. In some other cases, during the first trial the animals
manifested intensive flexions of the body with temporal rhythmic fore- or
hindlimb movement, accompanied by 8 Hz RSA. However, all these very
intensive movements dissappeared during consecutive trials on the following
days, and RSA of 8 Hz or more was observed only during the rhythmical
hindlimbs movement.

Rhythmical movements of the hindlimbs evoked by rhythmical pressure in
plantar region were either accompanied by desynchronized EEG or by short-
lasting episodes of RSA up to 7 HZ, and never above that.

DISCUSSION

The lack of synchrony in the dorsal hippocampal activity recorded
during passive movement of the hindlimbs supports the view that hippocampal
RSA does not depend on proprioceptive feedback (Klemm 1972 et al.).

It is of interest that gross behavioral changes (e.g., locomotion) in
consecutive stages of instrumental training, are reflected in a relatively
narrow range of RSA frequency. The present data are consistent with other
findings on the narrow RSA frequency ranges on rats (Pickenhain and
Klingberg 1967) and cats (Elazar and Adey 1967).

The present study also suggests that full quadrupedal locomotion as
well as its reduced form, i.e., bipedal locomotion may be accompanied by
the same frequency of RSA. It may indicate that mechanisms of RSA depend
mainly on the elaboration of information from the external environment,
being independent of centrally programmed and actually performed movement.

Our claim is, however, in contradiction with the data obtained by Black and Young (1972), showing that the 'automatic' movements (e.g., licking), when utilized in both avoidance and appetitive instrumental conditioning procedure, are not accompanied by higher frequency RSA but the one below 7 Hz, which is typical of 'automatic' movements.

Locomotion of different velocity is known to result in change within a higher (7-12 Hz) range of RSA under certain conditions, whereas licking, which is always performed with constant frequency, is always accompanied by either RSA below 7Hz, or desynchronized EEG. For this reason it remains the same in instrumental training as during 'automatic' motor performance.

In conclusion: RSA frequency shift may help to differentiate between 'automatic' and 'volitional' movements in tests involving learning processes.

Acknowledgments

This investigation was supported by Projects 10.4.01.6 and 06.9.01.2 of the Polish Academy of Sciences. Special thanks are due to Mr S. Glazewski for collaborative efforts and Mrs K. Koperska for technical assistance.

REFERENCES

Black, A. H. and Young, G. A., 1972, Constraints on the operant conditioning of drinking, in: "Reinforcement: Behavioral Analyses," R. M. Gilbert and J. R. Millenson, eds., Academic Press, New York.

Elazar, Z. and Adey, W. R., 1967, Spectral analysis of low-frequency components in the electrical activity of the hippocampus during learning, Electroenceph.clin.Neurphysiol., 11:409.

Klemm, W. R., 1972, Effects of electric stimulation of brain stem reticular formation on hippocampal theta rhythm and muscle activity in unanesthetized, cervical- and midbrain transected rats, Brain Res., 41:331.

Korczyński, R., 1986, A simple device for measurement of escape-approach motivations (submitted for publication).

Korczyński, R. and Kasicki, S., 1986, Hippocampal RSA and hindlimb EMG activity in freely moving rat (submitted for publication).

Pickenhain, L. and Klingberg, F., 1967, Hippocampal slow-wave activity as a correlate of basic behavioral mechanisms in the rat, in: "Progress in Brain Research," W. R. Adey and T. Tokizane, eds., Elsevier, Amsterdam.

Whishaw, I. Q. and Vanderwolf, C. H., 1973, Hippocampal EEG and behavior: changes in amplitude and frequency of RSA (theta rhythm) associated with spontaneous and learned movement patterns in rats and cats, Behav.Biol., 8:461.

HIGHER DISTURBANCES OF MOVEMENT IN MONKEYS

(MACACA FASCICULARIS)

U. Halsband*

Department of Experimental Psychology
University of Oxford
Oxford, U.K.

Flexibility in being able to perform the appropriate action to the external situation constitutes a necessary condition for survival; without this ability the animal and man would fail to adjust to the specific demands of their external environment. But little is known of the brain mechanisms that allow the animal and man to choose the appropriate movement according to the external situation with which they are presented. There are neurological patients with damage to the frontal cortex who have great difficulty in carrying out purposeful movements without paralysis or a primary motor defect (normal strength, reflexes, coordination). Liepmann (1900) first described patients with lesions that included the frontal lobe and who demonstrated an inability to execute sequences of movements. He termed this deficit 'apraxia'. But although apraxia following frontal lobe damage was reported by many investigators (e.g., Botez, 1974; Denny-Brown, 1958; Kolb and Milner, 1981), it has not yet proved possible to identify a critical region in the frontal cortex in the work with patients. This is due to the fact that cortical damage in patients rarely affects a single functional or anatomical entity of the brain; consequently, it is difficult to correlate a particular deficit with the loss of a particular structure or area. Therefore in the present study higher movement disorders were investigated in a species where the experimenter can make surgical lesions in precisely defined regions of the frontal cortex.

Both the premotor cortex (area 6, also referred to as 'non-primary motor cortex' (Wise, 1984)) and the supplementary motor area are in a position to exert an influence on the primary motor cortex (area 4) via direct cortico-cortical paths (Künzle, 1978; Muakkassa and Strick, 1979). There is evidence that cortical association area direct their influence on area 4 via the premotor cortex and supplementary motor area (Bowker and Coulter, 1982; Petrides and Pandya, 1984). The prestriate and infero-temporal cortex send connections to area 8, and it is possible that they could influence the dorsal premotor cortex by connections from area 8 to area 6 (Arikuni et al., 1980; Godschalk et al., 1984). To perform a complex action, the motor cortex must ack on instructions from other areas on such crucial matters as i) which movement to choose; ii) which hand to use; iii) in which order to perform the movements and iv) where to move the hand in space.

_____
*Present address: Physiologisches Institut, Universität Kiel, Olshausenstraße 40, D-2300 Kiel 1, West Germany.

Eight adolescent cynomolgus monkeys (Macaca fascicularis) were faced
with a task in which an arbitrary visual cue (a color) specified the movement the animal had to perform. Preoperatively, the animals were trained
to push a vertical colored plaque to the left to uncover a hole in a per-
spex screen through which the animal could reach a vertical handle. They
were taught to pull a handle towards them when shown a blue plaque, and to
rotate it anticlockwise when shown a yellow cue. On any trial, either the
blue or the yellow plaque was presented, the order being determined by use
of the Gellerman schedule (Halsband and Passingham, in press). Operations
were performed on five of the animals, the remaining three monkeys serving
as unoperated controls; all ablations were bilateral. In three animals the
premotor cortex was removed including the posterior bank of the arcuate
sulcus, but not including the supplementary motor area. In two animals the
tissue of area 8 was removed including the frontal eye-fields. Figure 1
shows a typical lesion of the premotor cortex (PM) and the frontal eye-
fields (FEF) as reconstructed onto standard diagrams of the lateral view
and of coronal sections. In general, the lesions were as intended; full
details are given by Halsband and Passingham (in press). After the operation the animals with premotor lesions failed to relearn the task in 1000
trials (Figure 2). By contrast, the animals with frontal eye-fields

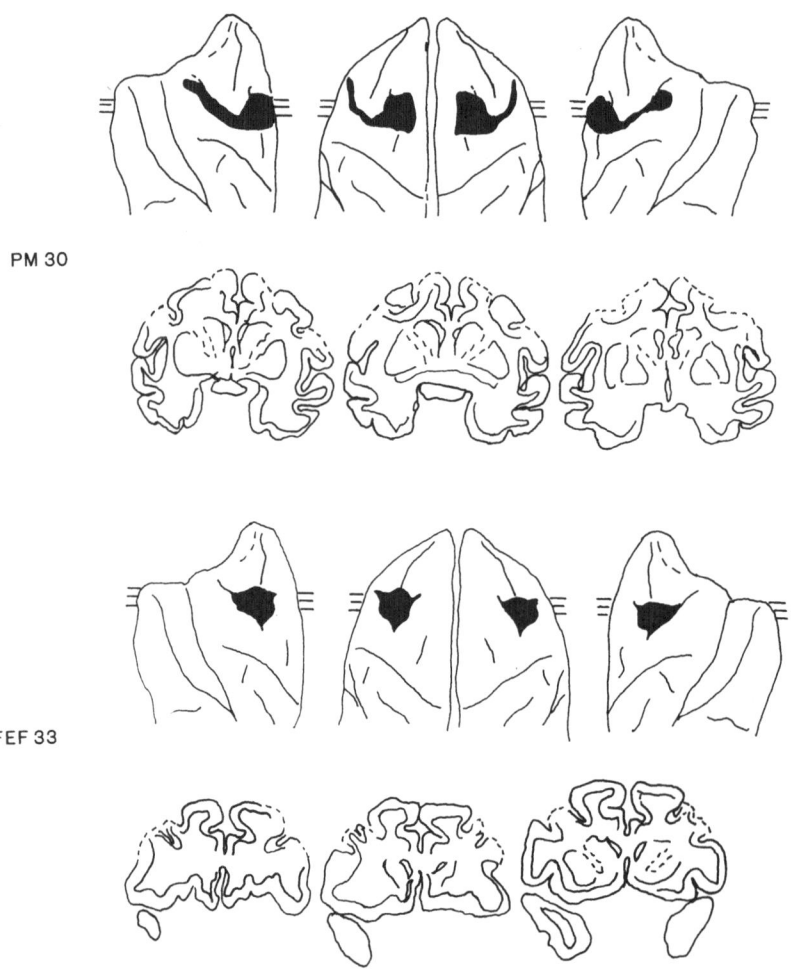

PM 30

FEF 33

Fig. 1. Reconstructions of the lesions of representative animals. PM =
         premotor; FEF = frontal eye-fields. The cross-sections were taken
         from the levels indicated by lines on the lateral views.

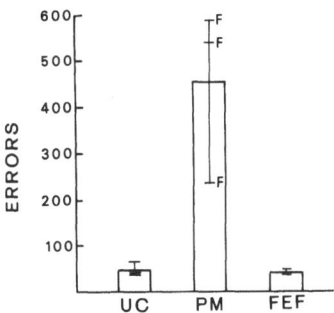

Fig. 2. Mean postoperative errors to criterion (180/200 trials correct) on the visual motor conditional task. Group PM failed to relearn the task after 1000 postoperative trials. The horizontal bars represent the errors for the individual animals.

lesions were not impaired and their errors did not differ from those of the animals that served as unoperated controls. The animals which could not master a task where they had to pull a handle when shown a blue cue and to turn it when shown a yellow cue also had difficulties in deciding which arm to use according to a visual instruction. Preoperatively the animals were taught to push a yellow cube with their preferred hand to to push with their non-preferred hand a red rod with a white stripe. On any trial one or other of these objects was present. The animal's task was to push the object so as to uncover a peanut, but given one object the animal must use its left hand and given another its right hand. In this task the animal has to make movements using the whole arm; a full description of the task is given by Halsband (1982). Figure 3 shows the postoperative errors made by the monkeys to reach criterion (180/200 trials correct). The animals with premotor lesions needed significantly more trials to re-learn this task than the unoperated control animals (p 0.05, two-tailed Mann-Whitney U test). The impairment on the conditional motor tasks after lesions of the premotor cortex is not the result of any simple motor or sensory defect. The monkeys had no trouble in learning a color discrimination nor in learning to make two new movements (Halsband and Passingham, 1982). They can also pick up objects between thumb and forefinger, deviate the wrist and supinate their forearm (Halsband, 1982); difficulties in these tasks occur with more extensive arcuate ablations (Moll and Kuypers, 1977; Halsband, 1982).

The question now arises whether the animals with premotor lesions have difficulties in choosing the appropriate action or whether these animals are generally impaired in making any choices according to a visual instruction. Postoperatively, the animals were trained on a visual conditional non-motor task (Halsband and Passingham, in press). The animal's task was to choose one of two objects: a brown wooden block or a white sphere. The animal first pushed a central panel and then made its choice: if the central panel was green the reward was to be found in a box that was covered by the white sphere, if the panel was orange it was to be found in a box that was covered by the brown block, the order being determined by use of the Gellerman schedule. From Figure 4 it can be seen that monkeys with premotor lesions can perform a visual conditional task so long as they are not required to select the appropriate movement according to the context. However, monkeys with lesions in the frontal eye-fields are impaired on this task: both animals failed to learn the conditional non-motor task in 3500 trials (Figure 4). Lawler (1981) has previously shown that monkeys with lesions in area 8 also have difficulties in using a central cue (black or white panel) to tell them whether food was to be found to the left or

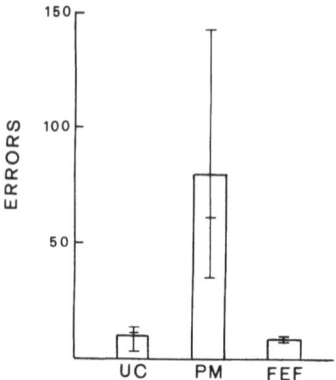

Fig. 3. Errors to relearn the conditional handedness task after the operation (180/200 trials correct).

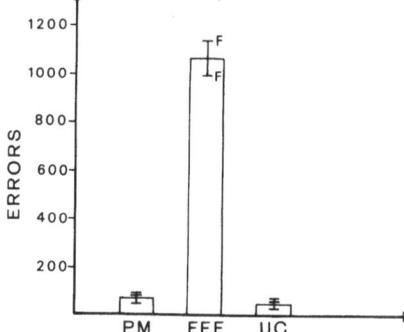

Fig. 4. Errors to criterion (180/200 trials correct) on a visual non-motor conditional task.

the right of the foodwell. Most recently Petrides (1985b) has shown that monkeys with lesions of the dorsal parts of areas 6 and 8 were impaired in learning a conditional non-motor task whereby the animal had to press a lit box given one cue and to press an unlit box given another. These findings point to a role of the frontal eye-fields in allowing the animal to pay sufficient attention to cues within peripheral vision.

The same animals with lesions in the premotor cortex which could not vary their movements as instructed by external cues were able to master a fixed three-sequence of movements to the same manipulandum where the cue for the second and third movements in the squence is the last movement (Halsband and Passingham, 1982). Passingham (1985) found that animals with combined lesions in both areas 6 and 8 were impaired in performing a sequence of three movements to three manipulanda positioned in different places. But this impairment may not be one of sequencing per se. Halsband (1982) trained monkeys on the spatial sequence task described by Passingham (1985) after the bilateral removal of either area 6 or 8 alone. Only the monkeys with lesions in area 8 were impaired in learning this task. It is likely that the animals with frontal eye-field ablations failed to learn the spatial sequences because they had difficulty in attending to different objects in space. Roland et al. (1981) measured cerebral blood flow while subjects performed a sequence of movements of the fingers. They found the supplementary motor cortex to be particularly active in the planning and execution of finger sequences. Orgogozo and Larsen (1979) similarly showed significant increases in local blood flow in the region of the supplementary motor cortex during complex sequential movement conditions. These results suggest a more specific involvement of the supplementary motor cortex in the programing of motor sequences. In line with these studies it is important to establish whether removal of cortex on the medial surface has any effect on the ability of a monky to perform a sequential task. In the following experiment therefore bilateral lesions were made in the supplementary motor area (n = 2). In two animals damage occurred to the medial frontal cortex anterior to the supplementary motor area. The animals with premotor ablations served as controls. Figure 5 shows cross-sections through the lesions of the four animals. Preoperatively, the animals were taught to push a T-shaped manipulandum upwards, then rotate it to the right and finally to hinge it up. The manipulandum returned to its original position after each movement. If the animals omitted one or more of the above movements the trial was terminated. Both animals with bilateral supplementary motor and one animal with medial frontal ablations were unable to re-learn the task after 1000 postoperative trials, the other animal needed 782 trials to re-meet criterion (180/200 correct trials) (Figure 6).

Taken together the present findings argue for distinct neurological mechanisms underlying movements and handedness discrimination versus the

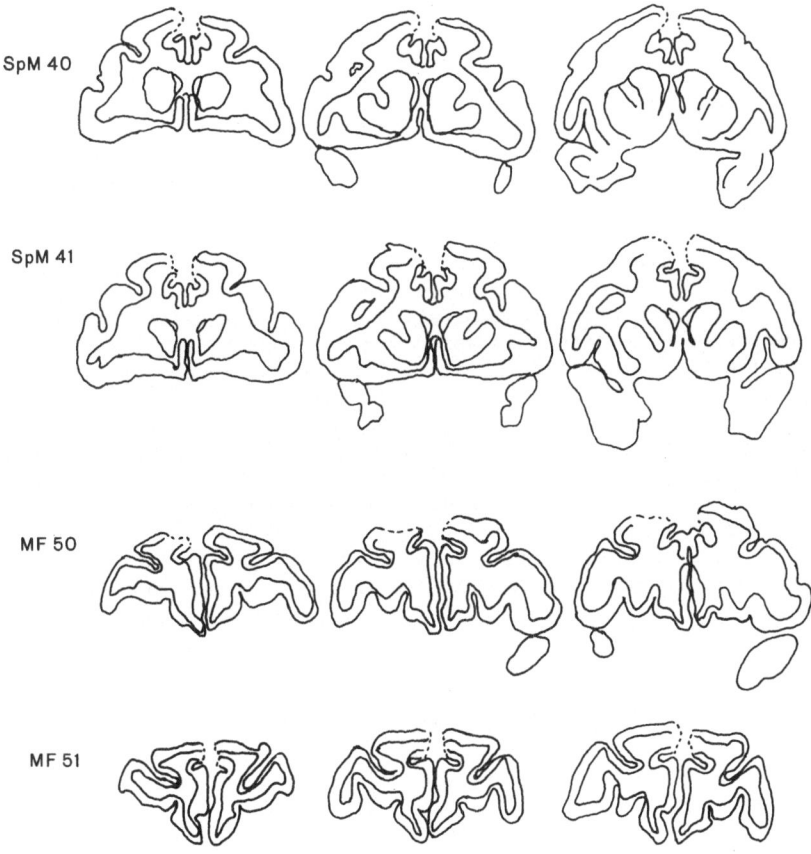

Fig. 5. Cross-sections through the supplementary motor (SpM) and medial frontal (MF) lesions. The dotted line indicates the area removed. In animal MF 50 post-mortem damage occurred to the frontal convexity.

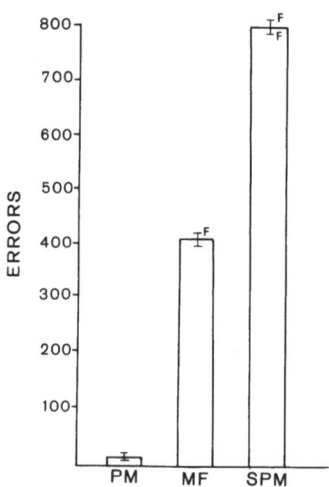

Fig. 6. Errors to relearn the three-sequence task after the operation
(180/200 trials correct). Both animals of Group SpM and one
animal of Group MF failed to relearn the task after 1000 postoperative trials.

animal's ability to perform complex sequences of movements or to visually
guide its hand in space:

i) The <u>premotor cortex</u> plays a crucial role in directing which movement
is to be made according to the external situation with which the
animals are presented. Most recently Petrides (1985a) reported that
patients with frontal lobe damage were impaired in learning to select
the correct movement to a given stimulus; it is possible that this
deficit was due to a disruption of the crucial influence the premotor
area seems to exert on the primary motor cortex. In both man and
monkey the impairment on the conditional tasks does not appear to be
due to difficulties in discriminating between the stimuli or in making
the responses, but rather in selecting the appropriate action.
ii) Medial frontal cortex and in particular the <u>supplementary motor area</u>
seem to be involved in the control of internally generated motor
sequences. Further experiments are needed to clarify whether the
supplementary motor area is critically involved in directly instruct-
ing the primary motor cortex in which order a given series of movements has to be performed or whether it is more generally involved in
the direction of actions.
iii) The <u>frontal eye-fields</u> seem to play a role in the direction of
attention in space. The present findings may be relevant for the
understanding of apraxia following frontal lobe damage in man.

Acknowledgments

I thank Dr R. E. Passingham for his invaluable advice with the design
of the experiments, Dr R. Saunders for performing the supplementary motor
ablations and Mrs H. C. Dawson for successfully typing the manuscript under
great pressure.

REFERENCES

Arikuni, T., Sakai, M., Hamada, J., and Kubota, K., 1980, Topographical
projections from the prefrontal cortex to the post-arcuate area in

the rhesus monkey, studied by retrograde axonal transport of horse-radish peroxidase, Neurosci.Lett., 19:155-160.

Botez, M. J., 1974, Frontal lobe tumours, in: "Handbook of Clinical Neurology," P. J. Vinken and G. W. Bruyk, eds., Elsevier/North-Holland, Amsterdam.

Bowker, R. M., and Coulter, J. D., 1981, Intracortical connectivities of somatic sensory and motor area: multiple cortical pathways in monkeys, in: "Cortical Sensory Organization," C. N. Woolsey, ed., Humana, Clifton, New Jersey.

Denny-Brown, D., 1958, The nature of apraxia, J.Nerv.Ment.Dis., 126:9-32.

Godschalk, M., Lemon, R. N., Kuypers, H. G. J. M., and Ronday, H. K., 1984, Cortical afferents and efferents of monkey postarcuate area: an anatomical and electrophysiological study, Exper.Brain Res., 56:410-424.

Halsband, U., 1982, "Higher Movements Disorders in Monkeys," Unpublished D.Phil. thesis, University of Oxford.

Halsband, U., and Passingham, R. E., 1982, The role of premotor and parietal cortex in the direction of action, Brain Res., 240:368-372.

Halsband, U., and Passingham, R. E., 1985, Premotor cortex and the conditions for movement in monkeys (Macaca fascicularis), Beh.Brain Res. (in press).

Kolb, R., and Milner, B., 1981a, Performance of complex arm and facial movements after focal brain lesions, Neuropsychologia, 19:491-504.

Künzle, H., 1978a, An autoradiographic analysis of the efferent connections from premotor and adjacent prefrontal regions (area 6 and 9) in Macaca fascicularis, Brain Beh.Evol., 15:185-234.

Lawler, K. A., 1981, Aspects of spatial vision after brain damage, Unpublished D.Phil. thesis, University of Oxford.

Liepmann, H., 1900, Das Krankheitsbild der Apraxie (motorischer Asymbolie), Monatsschr.Psychiatr., 8:15-44; 102-132; 183-197.

Moll, L., and Kuypers, H. G. J. M., 1977, Premotor cortical ablations in monkeys: contralateral changes in visually guided reaching behaviour, Science, 198:317-319.

Muakkassa, K. F., and Strick, P. L., 1979, Frontal lobe inputs to primate motor cortex: evidence for four somatotopically organized 'premotor' areas, Brain Res., 177:176-182.

Orgogozo, J. M., and Larsen, B., 1979, Activation of the supplementary motor area during voluntary movement in man suggests it works as a supramotor area, Science, 206:847-850.

Passingham, R. E., 1985, Prefrontal cortex and the sequencing of movement in monkeys (Macaca mulatta), Neuropsychologia, 23:453-462.

Petrides, M., 1985a, Deficits on conditional associative-learning tasks after frontal - and temporal - lobe lesions in man, Neuro-psychologia, 23:601-614.

Petrides, M., 1985b, Deficits in non-spatial conditional associative learning after periarcuate lesions in the monkey, Behav.Brain Res., 16:95-107.

Petrides, M., and Pandya, D. N., 1984, Projections to the frontal cortex from the posterior parietal region in the rhesus monkey, J.Comp. Neurol., 228:105-116.

Roland, P. E., Meyer, E., Shibasaki, T., Yamamoto, Y. L., and Thompson, C. J., 1982, Regional cerebral blood flow changes in cortex and basal ganglia during voluntary movements in normal human volunteers, J.Neurophysiol., 48:467-480.

Wise, S. P., 1984, The nonprimary motor cortex and its role in the cerebral control of movement, in: "Dynamic Aspects of Neocortical Function," G. Edelman, W. Gall, and W. Coward, eds., Wiley, New York.

CHARACTERISTICS OF DENTATE NEURONAL DISCHARGE IN A

SIMPLE AND A CHOICE REACTION TIME TASK IN THE MONKEY

C. E. Chapman* and Y. Lamarre

Centre de Recherche en Sciences Neurologiques and
*Ecole de Réadaptation, Université de Montréal
Montréal, Canada

A role for the lateral cerebellar system (hemisphere and dentate nucleus) in the planning, initiation and execution of movement is suggested by its connectivity: it receives input from the associative regions of cerebral cortex and projects to the precentral motor cortical areas (Allen and Tsukahara, 1974). In a recent study, we found that the discharge of dentate neurons, occurring well in advance of movement, does not specify the subsequent direction of movement in a simple reaction time (RT) task (Chapman et al., 1986). This is in marked contrast to, for example, motor cortex where the large majority of neurons, in this same task, are directional (Lamarre et al., 1980, 1981, 1983). It was, furthermore, difficult to reconcile these observations with those of other investigators who have reported a large proportion of direction-sensitive responses in dentate (Thach, 1970; Harvey et al., 1979; Stein, 1978; cf. Thach et al., 1982). It was suggested that the relative absence of direction-dependent discharge in this previous study might be explained by nature of the task used - a simple RT situation, with no preparatory period, in which the GO signal did not specify the desired direction of movement.

In order to investigate this question further, we have compared the results obtained from the 2 monkeys trained to perform the previously used simple RT task (Chapman et al., 1986) with those obtained in a third monkey trained to perform the same elbow movements in a choice RT task in which the GO signal also indicated the desired direction of movement. This same monkey was subsequently trained to perform a simple RT task in which the GO signal did not indicate the direction of movement. The latter task differed from our original simple RT task in that only a single stimulus, rather than three stimuli of different modalities, was used to signal movement.

Details of the task and the methods for data collection and analysis have been described elsewhere (Lamarre et al., 1983). For the choice RT task, one monkey (m. mulatta) was trained to perform a rapid flexion of the elbow in response to a tone of 400 Hz and a rapid extension of the elbow to a tone of 1000 Hz. The two tones were randomly presented to the monkey and

*Correspondance to: Dr C. E. Chapman, Centre de Recherche en Sciences Neurologiques, Faculté de Médecine, Université de Montréal, P.O. Box 6128, Station A, Montréal, Québec, Canada H3C 3J7.

the subsequent movements of flexion and extension were approximately symmetrical. Following training, a chamber was implanted over the cerebral hemisphere ipsilateral to the trained arm. Recordings were made from the dentate nucleus during the performance of the task. Following this series of recordings, the same monkey was subsequently retrained to perform blocks of flexions or extensions of the elbow in response to a single tone of 800 Hz (simple RT task). The desired direction of movement was indicated by only rewarding movements in the correct sense as in our previous study (Chapman et al., 1986). A series of recordings were then made, from the same regions of dentate as were sampled previously.

A total of 99 cells were recorded in the dentate nucleus (45 cells during the complex RT task and 54 cells during the simple RT task). Figure 1 shows examples of the types of responses recorded in these tasks. In contrast to our previous study, discharge before the onset of displacement was frequently directional, in both the complex and the simple RT task. Of the cells showing a clear modulation prior to movement onset in the complex RT task (n=26), the discharge pattern of 42% (11/26) varied, in a nonreciprocal fashion, with the subsequent direction of movement while the remainder (15/26) were nondirectional. Reciprocal changes (increase for one direction and decrease for the opposite direction) in discharge were never seen prior to the onset of movement. For the cell shown in Figure 1 (top), for example, the discharge increased 30 ms after the cue signaling a flexion movement (200 ms prior to the onset of displacement of the elbow). Following the cue for extension, however, there was no obvious modulation of discharge at the same latency. For both directions of movement, discharge increased during the movement, the increase ending at the turning point of the movement. This particular cell was not obviously directional during the movement but the majority of units (63%) demonstrated some form of direction-sensitivity during movement and this was occasionally reciprocally organized (one-quarter of the direction-sensitive units).

In the simple RT task, the discharge pattern of 32% (n=6) of the cells which were clearly modulated prior to movement (n=19) was directional. As was the case for the choice RT task, reciprocal discharge patterns were never seen prior to the onset of movement. The majority of cells (68%) had a nondirectional discharge pattern prior to the onset of movement. An example of this is shown in Figure 1 (bottom). This cell showed an increase in discharge, beginning 80 ms after the two cues; the magnitude and timing of the increase was the same for the two directions of movement. During movement, a reciprocal pattern of discharge was observed: a decrease in discharge during extension and an increase in discharge during the flexion movements. In general, the discharge of 79% (15/19) of the dentate neurons was directional during movement in this simple RT task, with about one-half of the cells (7/15) showing a reciprocal pattern of discharge.

In a simple RT task requiring that the animal attend three different, randomly presented cues (a tone, a light and a small, brief perturbation applied to the operant forearm), we found that few dentate neurons showed evidence of direction-dependence prior to the onset of movement (Chapman et al., 1986). Only 10% of the cells tested were direction-sensitive prior to movement, none of these showing a reciprocal pattern of discharge. While the proportion of direction-sensitive cells was greater during, as compared to before, movement (31% vs. 10%) in our original task, this was still much lower than the proportions found here in the complex (63%) and simple (79%) RT tasks. Furthermore, the proportion of reciprocal to nonreciprocal cells was changed - reciprocal responses were 2 to 4 times more frequently observed in these tasks as compared to the original task.

CHOICE REACTION TIME

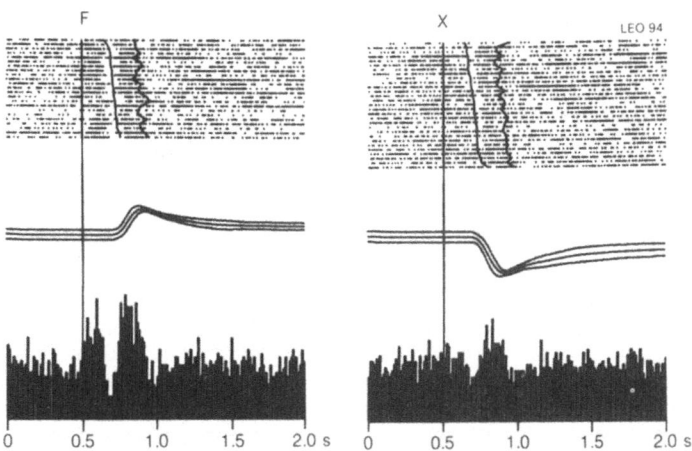

SIMPLE REACTION TIME

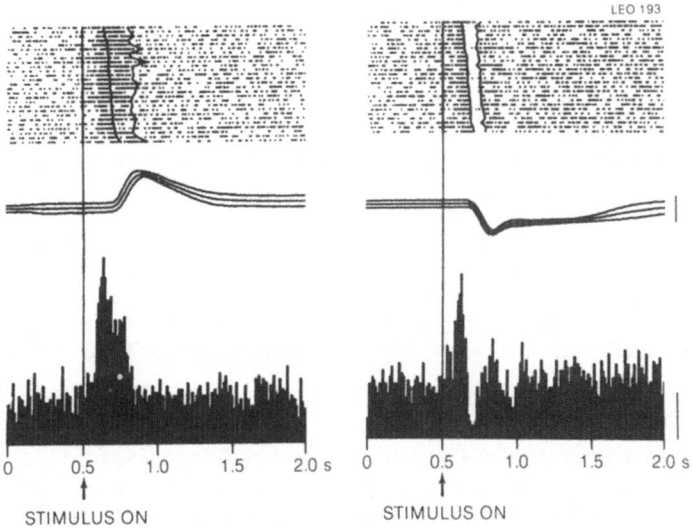

STIMULUS ON   STIMULUS ON

Fig. 1.   Activity of two dentate neurons during flexion (F) and extension
(X) of the ipsilateral elbow. Above: typical response of a neuron
recorded during the choice RT task.   Direction-sensitive discharge
preceded the onset of movement (indicated by the first of two
irregular lines running through each raster) and was followed by,
in this case, a nonspecific (i.e., nondirectional) increase in
discharge during movements in the two directions. The late increase in discharge ended at the turning point of the movement
(shown as the second irregular line running through the raster).
Below: response of a dentate neuron recorded during the simple RT
task (one tone).   This unit showed a symmetrical increase in
discharge prior to the onset of movement in the two directions.
For the flexion movements, the increase continued until the time
of peak deceleration (second irregular line).   For the extension
movements, the increase ended at the onset of movement and was
followed by a decrease in discharge, ending at the time of peak
velocity (second irregular line), i.e., there was a reciprocal
response pattern during movement.   All rasters are aligned on the
presentation of the stimulus and the trials have been rearranged
(cont'd on next page)

in order of increasing reaction time. The movement traces represent an average of all trials shown in the corresponding raster (±1 S.D. of the mean). The vertical calibration bars represent 50 degrees (movement) and 50 impulses/sec (unit firing rate).

←——

A further difference between the results of these two studies is that there was a large change in the proportion of stimulus- to movement-related cells (analysis based upon the timing of the initial change in discharge, preceding movement). In the original study, stimulus-related cells were three times more frequently encountered than movement-related cells. Excluding those cells in which there was only a response to the visual or the somesthetic cue, stimulus-related cells would still have been expected to be more than twice as frequent as movement-related cells in this study. But, the proportions were reversed here: movement-related cells were 2 to 3 times more frequently encountered than stimulus-related cells. Preliminary results indicate that differences in the task may explain the difference between these results. The same monkey was retrained a second time, to respond to a visual as well as the auditory cue. While only a few cells were recorded in this situation (n=29), the results were similar to those obtained in our original study: the proportions of direction-dependent responses were much lower prior to and during movement and there were relatively more stimulus- than movement-related responses.

In conclusion, no real differences in dentate discharge character-istics were seen when comparing the results obtained from one monkey trained to perform the same movements in two different situations. Discharge was frequently directional and time-locked to the performance of the movement in both complex and simple RT situations. The results were, however, very different from those obtained in monkeys trained to perform similar movements in response to three different sensory cues, each of a different modality. Preliminary results suggest that the cerebellar dentate nucleus may play a special role in situations in which the animal must simultaneously attend more than one sensory modality.

Acknowledgments

The authors gratefully acknowledge the assistance provided by the technical staff of the Centre de recherche en sciences neurologiques, and in particular by M. T. Parent, R. Bouchoux, S. Bergeron, and P. Aubrey. This research was supported by a Medical Research Council of Canada group grant. C. E. Chapman is a scholar of the Fonds de la recherche en santé du Québec. Y. Lamarre is a member of the Canadian MRC Group in Neurological Sciences.

REFERENCES

Allen, G. I., AND Tsukahara, N., 1974, Cerebrocerebellar communication systems, Physiol.Rev., 54:957-1006.
Chapman, C. E., Spidalieri, G., and Lamarre, Y., 1986, Activity of dentate neurons during arm movements triggered by visual, auditory and somesthetic stimuli in the monkey, J.Neurophysiol. (in press).
Harvey, R. J., Porter, R., and Rawson, J. A., 1979, Discharges of intra-cerebellar nuclear cells in monkeys, J.Physiol.(Lond.), 297:559-580.
Lamarre, Y., Spidalieri, G., Busby, L., and Lund, J. P., 1980, Programming of initiation and execution of ballistic arm movements in the monkey, in: "Progress in Brain Research. Motivation, Motor and Sensory Processes of the Brain," H. H. Kornhuber and L. Deecke, eds., Elsevier/North Holland Biomedical Press, Amsterdam.

Lamarre, Y., Spidalieri, G., and Chapman, C. E., 1983, A comparison of neuronal discharge recorded in the sensori-motor cortex, parietal cortex and dentate nucleus of the monkey during arm movements triggered by light, sound or somesthetic stimuli, Exp.Brain Res. Suppl., 7:140-156.

Lamarre, Y., Spidalieri, G., and Lund, J. P., 1981, Patterns of muscular and motor cortical activity during a simple arm movement in the monkey, Can.J.Physiol.Pharmacol., 59:748-756.

Stein, J., 1978, Long loop motor control in monkeys. The effects of transient cooling of parietal cortex and of cerebellar nuclei during tracking tasks, in: "Progress in Clinical Neurophysiology. Cerebral Motor Control in Man: Long Loop Mechanisms," J. E. Desmedt, ed., Karger, Basel.

Thach, W. T., 1970, Discharge of cerebellar neurons related to two maintained postures and two prompt movements, I. Nuclear cell output, J.Neurophysiol., 33:527-536.

Thach, W. T., Perry, J. G., and Schieber, M. H., 1982, Cerebellar output: body maps and muscle spindles, Exp.Brain Res.Suppl., 6:440-454.

MOVEMENT RELATED BRAIN POTENTIALS IN

SUSTAINED ISOMETRIC VOLUNTARY CONTRACTION

B. Dimitrov, G. N. Gantchev, and D. Popivanov

Institute of Physiology
Bulgarian Academy of Sciences
Sofia, Bulgaria

INTRODUCTION

The potentials preceding a volitional act, namely the BEREITSCHAFTS-POTENTIAL (Deecke et al., 1969) and the accompanying components (Vaughan et al., 1968) have been extensively analyzed. Whatever happens at the end of a prolonged voluntary act, however, is still far from clear. Weinberg (1980) found a potential at the moment of self-stopped guided movement and Ivanova (1984) at voluntary termination of a movement. We have chosen the sustained isometric contraction as a model representing a complex act of initiation and termination of an effort. We have confirmed the presence of Movement Related Brain Potentials (MRBPs) at the end of the sustained contraction, similar to MRBPs at the beginning of contraction (Gantchev et al., 1982). The possible influence of a sustained positivity throughout maintained effort (Otto et al., 1977, Grünewald-Zuberbier et al., 1980) was ruled out by producing negative potentials at the moment of an additional press superimposed upon a maintained isometric effort (Gantchev and Dimitrov, 1983).

To exclude the possible role of the antagonists' involvement at the moment of the sharp relaxation of sustained contraction we attempted to compare movements with similar beginning and different termination and movements with different beginning and similar termination around one particular joint. It turned out that the negativity was not influenced by the type of the movement and, consequently, MRBPs could be associated with a relaxation command (Dimitrov, 1985). Now, in pursuit for a simple agonist-antagonist interaction we selected the pair of arm biceps/triceps muscles. The biceps isometric contraction was chosen as a basic voluntary act, performed once solitary and, secondly, with concomitant cocontraction of triceps. Brain potentials related to both the beginning and termination of isometric effort were obtained and compared.

METHODS

The subjects were seated in an armchair providing comfortable support for the right elbow. In the first task they performed abrupt isometric contraction of the biceps, maintained at a steady level for about 3 seconds and terminated without triceps involvement. In the second task the isometric cocontraction of both biceps and triceps was required. The EMG was recorded via surface bipolar electrodes placed over the lateral ridge of the respective muscles, differentially amplified and bandpass filtered (10-2 KHz) by using electromyograph MEDICOR MG 42. Both EMGs were fed to separate channels of a video terminal VM 61/A placed in front of the subject so that he could control the full relaxation of the muscles before each trial, the inactivity of triceps during simple biceps contraction and the sharp edges of the rise and fall of the EMG activity utilizing this visual feedback. Several training sessions were conducted until satisfactory performance had been reached. The two tasks, each comprising 36 contraction/relaxation trials were repeated twice in the experiment involving 5 subjects.

5 scalp electrodes BECKMAN were positioned at F_3, C_3, P_3, FC_z and C_z (FC_z being the mid-distance between F_z and C_z) attached with adhesive paste and referenced to linked earlobe clips. The EOG was monitored via bipolar upper and lateral orbital ridge skin electrodes BECKMAN. An 8 channel ALVAR TR 6 electroencephalograph was set at bandpass 0.026 - 70 Hz and EEG and EMG data were collected together in the computer MINC 23 (DEC, USA) on-line (A/D converter sampling intervals 11 ms, resolution of 12 bits).

A software procedure was invented for single trial MRBP preprocessing which was applied off-line. It included a subroutine for detection of single trial EMG edges (the start of contraction and the start of relaxation) and the shifting of EEG records so that their longer part preceded the detected starts. Then each EEG segment was fitted once to the EMG ascending edge and secondly to the EMG descending edge. The EMG edges were detected by using an iterative procedure on the basis of comparison of the cummulative sums of the rectified EMG segments preceding and following the time point detected by an appropriately chosen threshold (Popivanov, 1986). This procedure was automated but the active participation of the experimenter was permitted in dialogue regime (Figure 1). Another subroutine was provided for visual inspection of a chosen EEG segment. If the EEG was considered artifact-free it was averaged, otherwise all EEG channels were erased.

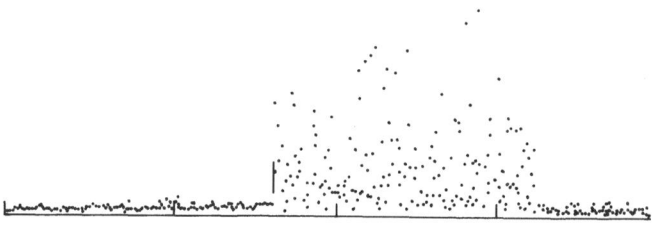

```
INITIAL  LEVEL  BOUNDARIES:  L1=, L2=
? 0
? 100
THRESHOLD:  T=
? 2
START  ADDRESS  TO  CHECK  FIRST SET-ON:  C=
? 150
NUMBER  OF  POINTS  FOR  AREA:
? 9
AREAS  RATIO:  A=
? 2
```

Fig. 1.   An example of the initial dialogue for determining the single trial EMG start (vertical bar). The trace duration is 5.5 s (500 samples, 11 ms sampling interval).

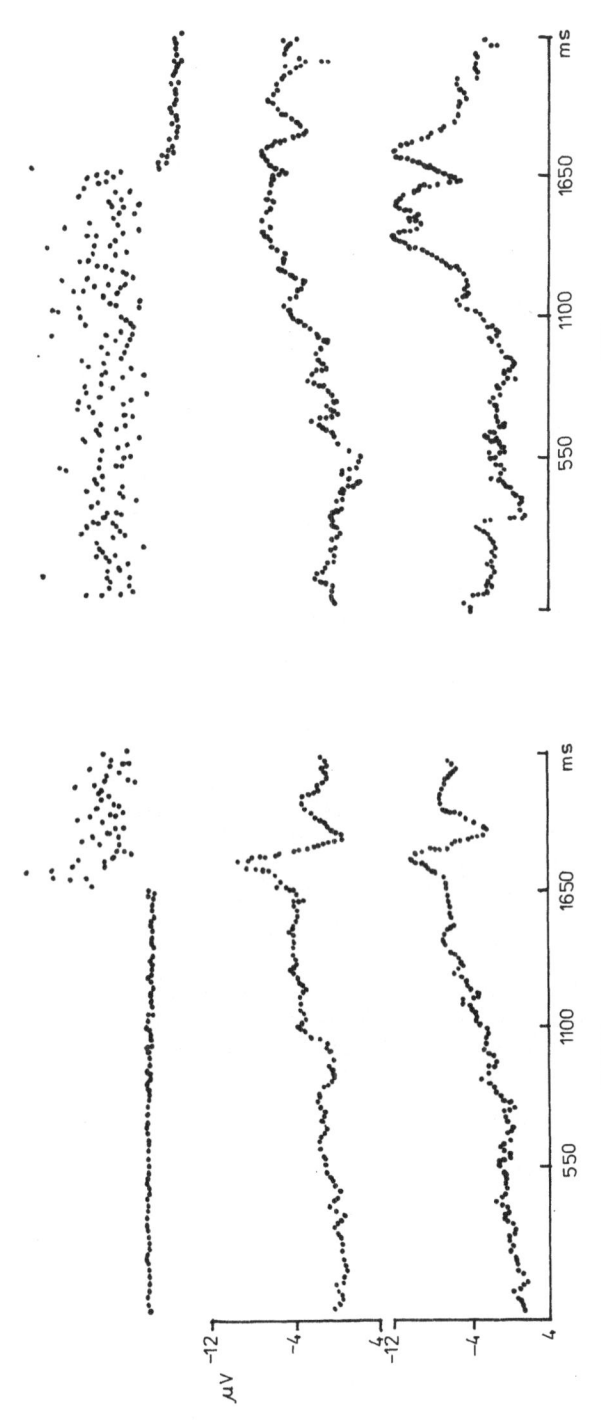

Fig. 2. Averaged Movement Related Brain Potentials aligned to the beginning (left columns) and to the termination (right columns) of a sustained isometric contraction. First row- averaged EMG. Second row-MRBPs in biceps contraction. Third row-MRBPs in biceps/triceps cocontraction.

The baseline of the averaged epoch of 1650 ms before and 550 ms after the start (resp. end) of the contraction/cocontraction was automatically estimated from the mean voltage of the first 220 ms and amplitude values at 150 ms preceding EMG edge (BP_{150}), at the start (end) of the effort (BP_0), maximal negativity (N_2) and maximal following positivity (P_2) were printed. The data were subjected to a two-way ANOVA statistics.

RESULTS

The two tasks of contraction/cocontraction starts and ends produced four distinguished concomitant MRBPs. They are presented in Figure 2 for one experimental subject. The data from ANOVA for the four measured parameters are presented in Table 1. The significant influence of both factor A (type of effort: A1 - contraction start, A2 - contraction end, A3 - cocontraction start, A4 - cocontraction end) and factor B (lead: F_3, C_3, P_3, FC_z, C_z) increased with consecutive measures of negativity approaching effort execution. The positivity did not differ among effort and lead.

F_d values for partial differences (Figure 3) revealed greater negativity for cocontraction start than simple contraction start, significantly higher negativity for both contraction/cocontraction starts compared to respective ends and, noteworthy, lack of difference between contraction and cocontraction ends. These features were unilaterally expressed for the three parameters BP_{150}, BP_0 and N_2. For P_2 measures only positivity following the beginning of sustained contraction was lesser than that following the end of both contraction and cocontraction.

The scalp distribution presented the well known maximum over the vertex (C_z), significantly higher than lateral positions F_3, C_3, P_3 for the early measurement BP_{150}. As the moment of action approached however, the lead over supplementary motor area (FC_z) turned out to be significantly lower than C_z and did not differ from lateral leads (measurements BP_0 and N_2). For these measurements, although greater than F_3 and P_3, FC_z amplitude did not differentiate from that over C_3 (motor area). Similar relationships were noted for P_2.

DISCUSSION

The pronounced prevalence of negative amplitudes preceding efforts of cocontraction compared to those of simple contraction is in view with the amount of negativity being proportional to the level of general facilitation. The cocontraction requires greater intentional involvement by the

Table 1. Two-Way ANOVA for MRBPs Amplitude Values

Source of variance	Degrees of freedom	F values				F.05	F.01
		BP_{150}	BP_0	N_2	P_2		
A	3	3.59*	9.05**	14.58**	1.85	2.70	3.98
B	4	3.10*	3.51*	7.56**	1.45	2.46	3.51
AxB	12	0.77	0.28	0.58	0.19	1.85	2.37
Mean	119						

A - type of effort.
B - lead.

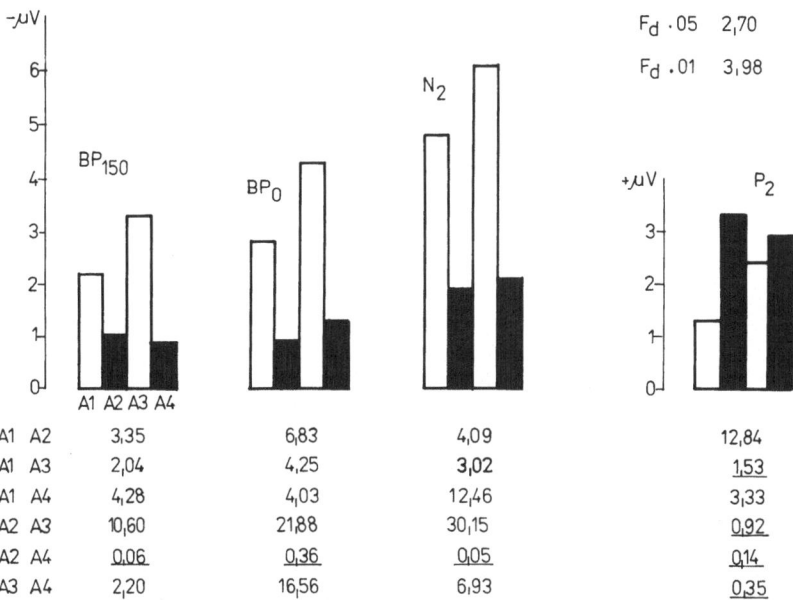

		BP$_{150}$	BP$_0$	N$_2$	P$_2$
A1	A2	3,35	6,83	4,09	12,84
A1	A3	2,04	4,25	3,02	1,53
A1	A4	4,28	4,03	12,46	3,33
A2	A3	10,60	21,88	30,15	0,92
A2	A4	0,06	0,36	0,05	0,14
A3	A4	2,20	16,56	6,93	0,35

Fig. 3.   Mean amplitudes of the four measured amplitudes of MRBPs. A1-
start, A2- end of sustained biceps contraction. A3- start, A4-
end of sustained biceps/triceps cocontraction. F$_d$ values for
partial differences derived from two-way ANOVA.

subject and the participation of more muscles is represented by augmented
differences toward the moment of the execution (BP$_{150}$ vs. BP$_0$&N$_2$). The
significant diminution of MRBPs at the moment of relaxation of both contraction and cocontraction compared to the starts has been already observed
in previous studies (Gantchev et al., 1982) and is probably due to the
influence of sustained positivity during sustained contraction (see Otto
et al., 1977). It should be underlined that there were no conditions
favoring negativity in this study (as in goal-directed movements,
Grünewald-Zuberbier et al., 1980) and the length of the maintained contraction did not exceed 3 seconds. The discordance with the phasic pronounced positivity described by Ivanova (1984) is somehow unexplainable,
probably due to the external cue employed in her study.

Most valuable is the fact that contraction and cocontraction relax-
ations were accompanied by virtually the same potentials (A2 vs. A4).
Although diminished in comparison to the corresponding start MRBPs (A1 vs.
A2 and A3 vs. A4) and although the preceding start MRBPs were different
among themselves (A1 vs. A3) it seems the relaxation was performed in a
state of equal excitation and cortical involvement, regardless of the
physical and psychological differences. We ought to be cautious, however,
drawing conclusions about cerebral generators by employing gross scalp
macropotential recordings. It is not clear if an inhibition command that
is present eventually could be verified and qualitatively estimated by
using this methodological approach.

What we are dealing with is, in fact, not registering certain switch-on/switch-off commands, but the intermediate result from the action of not-well restricted areas. Thus the only positive conclusion would be that there is no difference in MRBPs accompanying the end of voluntary action which depend upon the particular background state and muscles involved and that these MRBPs are not a product of antagonists' involvement. In brief, we can support for the time being, the existence of a MRBP correlated with a command for relaxation.

REFERENCES

Deecke, L., Scheidt, P., and Kornhuber, H. H., 1969, Distribution of readiness potential, pre-motor positivity and motor potential of the human cerebral cortex preceding voluntary movement, Exp.Brain Res., 7:158.

Dimitrov, B., 1985, Brain potentials related to the beginning and to the termination of voluntary flexion and extension in man, Int.J. Psychophysiol., 3:13.

Gantchev, G. N., and Dimitrov, B., 1983, Brain potentials related to additional isometric contraction, Activ.nerv.sup.(Praha), 25:285.

Gantchev, G. N., Popivanov, D., and Dimitrov, B., 1982, Brain potentials related to voluntary sustained effort, Acta physiol.et pharmacol. bulg., 8:14.

Grünewald-Zuberbier, E., Grünewald, G., Schuhmacher, H., and Wehler, A., 1980, Scalp recorded slow potential shifts during isometric ramp and hold contractions in human subjects, Pflügers Archiv., 389:55.

Ivanova, M. P., 1984, Cortical motor potentials connected with voluntary termination of a movement, Zh.visch.nervn.de'yateln., (Russian), 34:437.

Otto, D. A., Benignus, V. A., Ryan, L. J., and Leiffer, L. J., 1977, Slow potential components of stimulus, response and preparatory processes in man. A multiple linear regression model, in: "Progress in Clinical Neurophysiology," vol.I, p.211, J. Desmedt, ed., S. Karger, Basel.

Popivanov, D., 1986, Computer detection of EMG edges for synchronization of Movement Related Brain Potentials, Electroenceph.clin.Neurophysiol. [1936, 64:171-176]

Vaughan, H. B., Costa, L. D., and Ritter, W., 1968, Topography of human motor potential, Electroenceph.clin.Neurophysiol., 25:1.

Weinberg, H., 1980, Slow potentials related to initiation and inhibition of proprioceptively guided movements, in: "Motivation, Motor and Sensory Processes of the Brain: Electrical Potentials, Behaviour and Clinical Use," Progress in Brain Res., vol.54, p.183, H. H. Kornhuber and L. Deecke, eds., Elsevier, Amsterdam.

ARE SELF-PACED REPETITIVE FATIGUING HAND CONTRACTIONS

ACCOMPANIED BY CHANGES IN MOVEMENT-RELATED BRAIN POTENTIALS?

G. Freude, P. Ullsperger, and M. Pietschmann

Central Institute of Occupational Medicine of the GDR
Department of Work Physiology
GDR

INTRODUCTION

Since the first publication on movement-related brain potentials (MRP) by Kornhuber and Deecke (1964, 1965), in investigations in this field have been extended considerably. There are a lot of experimental data from the analysis of the different components of the MRP and their physiological significance (Gerbrandt, 1977, Shibasaki et al., 1980, Deecke et al., 1976), on the connection between somatotopic organization and MRP (Vaughan, 1968), on the topographic distribution of MRP over the scalp (Deecke and Kornhuber, 1977, Gerbrandt, 1977, Vaughan, 1968, Shibasaki et al., 1980) etc.

It has been suggested that the Bereitschaftspotential (Bp) as the main component of the pre-movement-related brain potentials reflects cortical processes associated with preparatory mechanisms of the motor act.

It could be shown that the Bp also depends on the muscular effort. Becker and Kristeva (1980) have found that the Bp amplitude is higher prior to large than prior to small isometric force deployments. It has been postulated that a greater negativity of the Bp reflects a higher level of activity of the underlying cortical structures. The present study was to investigate the dependence of the Bp on the degree of muscular fatigue. There are many experimental data on changes of peripheral physiological parameters due to muscular fatigue, but little is known about simultaneous processes in the CNS.

METHOD

Six healthy right-handed subjects were instructed to rapidly squeeze a handgrip dynamometer with about 70% of maximal voluntary contraction (MVC) intermittently as long as possible self-paced at irregular intervals of about 4-10 sec.

Non-polarizing Ag/AgCl electrodes were placed over central areas C'_3 (1 cm anterior to C_3), C'_4 (1 cm anterior to C_4), C_z and linked ear electrodes served as common reference. Electrode impedances were less than 5 kOhm. Right supra- and infra-orbital electrodes were used to record the vertical electrooculogram (EOG). The EEGs, the EOG (time constant of 5 s, upper frequency cutoff 15 Hz) and the EMG of forearm muscles were amplified and, together with the force transducer signal, recorded on a 14-channel tape recorder. The arrangement of the experiment is shown in Figure 1.

The EEG signals were averaged time-locked to the onset of the movement (dynamometer output) 3000 ms prior to and 1000 ms afterwards, by means of a multichannel analyzer DIDAC 4000 at a 10-ms sampling rate. As there are interindividual differences in the total frequency of movements, the whole experimental period was divided into three equal stages.

The following parameters of Bp were measured by means of a lab computer: the areas of four equal 500-ms time intervals of the Bp (2000 ms – 1500 ms, 1500 ms – 1000 ms, 1000 ms – 500 ms, and 500 ms – 0 ms i.e., movement onset).

The areas of the four different Bp time intervals were tested by 3-factorial analyses of variance (subject, stage, electrode position) and multiple comparisons of mean values. The level of significance was set to 5%.

RESULTS

Figure 2 shows the mean movement-related brain potentials across all subjects for the first (——) and the last (---) experimental stage. The main finding, i.e., a higher, and earlier Bp prior to this movement in the

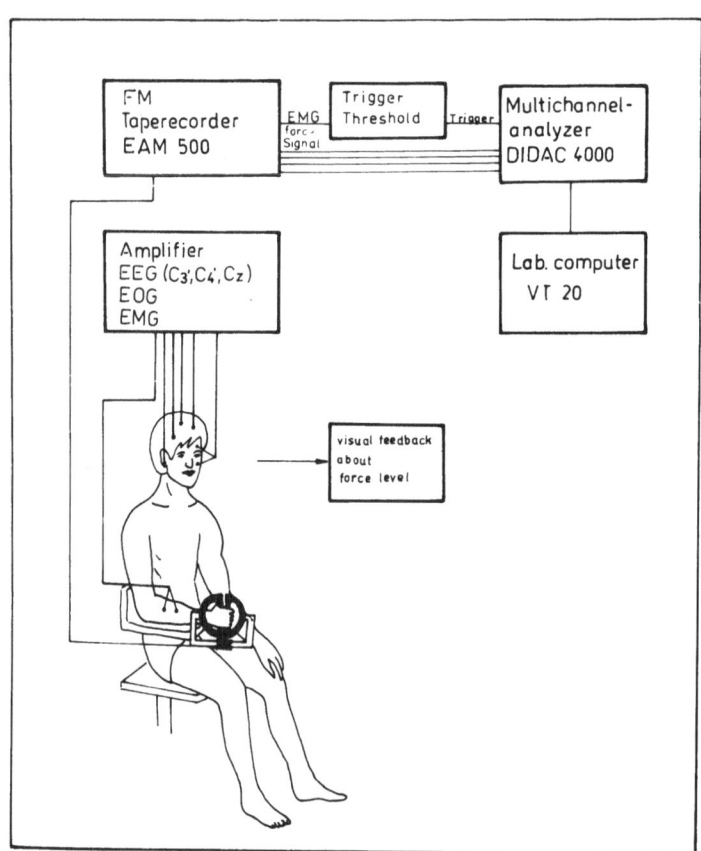

Fig. 1. Experimental arrangement.

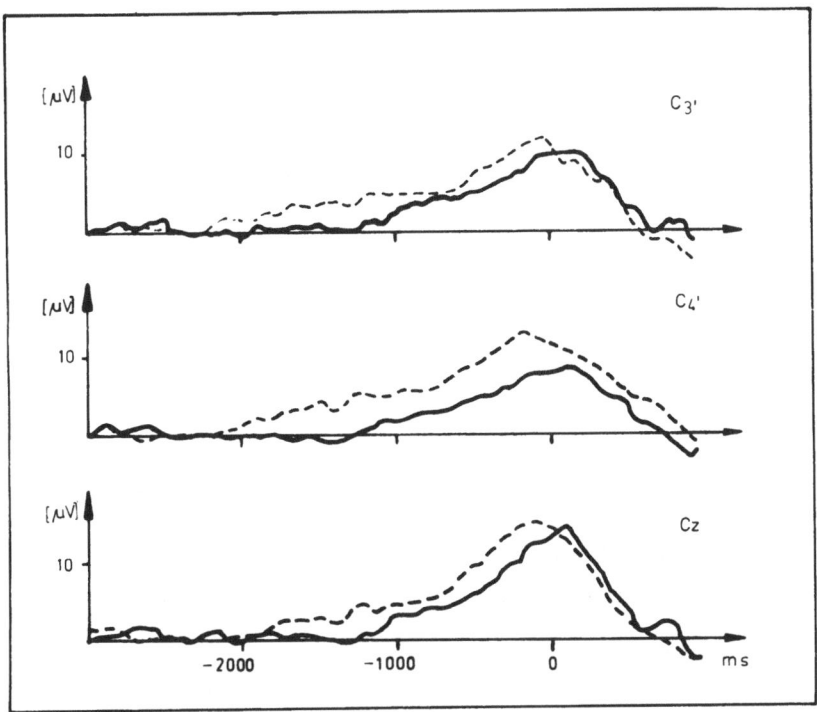

Fig. 2.   Grand averages of movement-related brain potentials.   0 indicates
          movement onset.   ——— mean waveform of the first experimental stage
          (1).   ——— mean waveform of the last experimental stage (3).

last experimental stage (the stage with the highest muscular fatigue)
compared with the Bp of the first experimental stage, is shown in this
figure. No significant differences in the Bp have been found between
stages 2 and 3.

Figure 3 shows the mean values of the areas of negativity of the Bp
for the four consecutive time intervals in the experimental stages 1 and 3.
Whereas for time intervals (2000 ms - 1500 ms) and (1500 ms - 1000 ms)
before the movement onset a small negativity was found in the first experimental stage, a considerable increase of the Bp activity occurred at these
time intervals in stage 3.

DISCUSSION

The present results show that muscular fatigue is accompanied by an
increased Bp. Related investigations on muscular fatigue and Bp have not
been found in literature. There are reports regarding changes of the Bp in
the course of non-fatiguing movements, only. For repetitive finger movements depending on the engagement or intentional involvement no changes or
a decrease of the Bp were observed by Kornhuber and Deecke (1964, 1965).
Becker and Kristeva (1980) reported that the Bp amplitude remained unchanged during an experimental phase with an average of 120 force deployments. The absence of a further increase between stages 2 and 3 in the
present experiment could be an effect of a decrease of engagement with the
increasing quantity of repetitive hand movements. Two different trends
with opposite directions may be assumed during fatiguing movements. The
greater negativity of Bp in the course of fatiguing hand contractions
possibly reflects a higher level of activity of the cortical structures

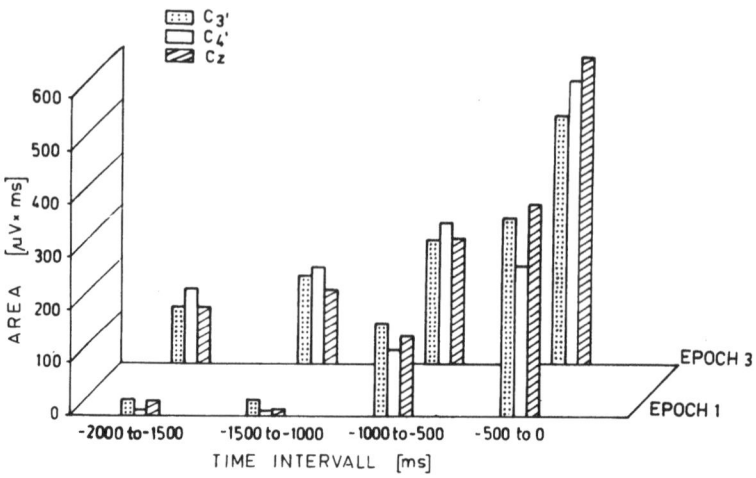

Fig. 3. Mean areas of negativity of the Bp at four consecutive time
intervals in stages 1 and 3. 0 indicates movement onset.

involved. It may be concluded that isometric hand contractions with
fatigued muscles involve a greater degree of cortical activation or in
other terms, the engagement must be higher when working with fatigued
muscles.

The increase of negativity from the experimental stages 1 to 3 was
more pronounced in the earlier phases of Bp. It is suggested that the
earlier phase of Bp (up to 500 ms before movement onset) reflects preparatory activity independent on the specific movement according to
Hillyard's (1973) two-component hypothesis (see also Kutas and Donchin,
1977, Shibasaki et al., 1980). Though the question of proper functional
significance of Bp remains open, it seems to be worthwhile to continue
investigations on Bp changes accompanying muscular fatigue to learn more
about central nervous mechanisms in the preparation of motor acts.

REFERENCES

Becker, W., and Kristeva, R., 1980, Cerebral potentials prior to various
        force deployments, Prog.Brain Res., 54:189.
Deecke, L., Grözinger, B., and Kornhuber, H. H., 1976, Voluntary finger
        movement in man: Cerebral potentials and theory, Biol.Cybern, 23:99.
Deecke, L., and Kornhuber, H. H., 1977, Cerebral potentials and the
        initiation of voluntary movement, in: "Attention, Voluntary Con-
        traction and Event-Related Cerebral Potentials," Progress in
        Clinical Neurophysiology, J. E. Desmedt, ed., Karger, Basel.
Gerbrandt, L. K., 1977, Analysis of movement potential components, in:
        "Attention, Voluntary Contraction and Event-Related Cerebral
        Potentials," Progress in Clinical Neurophysiology, J. E. Desmedt,
        ed., Kargar, Basel.
Hillyard, S. A., 1973, The CNV and human behavior, in: "Event-related Slow
        Potentials," W. C. McCallum and J. R. Knott, eds., Elsevier,
        Amsterdam-New York.

Kornhuber, H. H., and Deecke, L., 1964, Hirnpotentialänderungen beim
    Menschen vor und nach Willkürbewegungen, dargestellt mit Magnet-
    bandspeicherung und Rückwärtsanalyse, Pflügers Arch., 281:52.
Kornhuber, H. H., and Deecke, L., 1965, Hirnpotentialänderungen bei
    Willkürbewegungen und passiven Bewegungen des Menschen: Bereit-
    schaftspotential und reafferente Potentiale, Plügers Arch., 284:1.
Kristeva, R., and Kornhuber, H. H., 1980, Cerebral potentials related to
    the smallest human finger movement, in: "Motivation, Motor and
    Sensory Processes of the Brain," H. H. Kornhuber and L. Deecke, ed.,
    Elsevier, Amsterdam-New York.
Kristeva, R., 1984, Bereitschaftspotential of Painists, Annals of the New
    York Academie of Sciences, 425:477.
Kutas, M., and Donchin, E., 1977, The effect of handiness, of responding
    hand, and of response force and the contralateral dominance of the
    readiness potential, in: "Attention, Voluntary Contraction and
    Event-Related Cerebral Potentials," Progress in Clinical Neuro-
    physiology, J. E. Desmedt, ed., Karger, Basel.
Shibasaki, H., Barret, G., Halliday, E., and Halliday, A. M., 1980,
    Components of the movement-related cortical potentials and their
    scalp topography, Electroenceph.Clin.Neurophysiol., 49:213.
Vaughan, H. G., Costa, J. D., and Ritter, W., 1968, Topography of the human
    motor potential, Electroenceph.Clin.Neurophysiol., 25:1.

EFFECTS OF ANTAGONIST ACTIVATION ON SENSATIONS OF MUSCLE FORCE

L. Jones and I. Hunter

Department of Neurology and Neurosurgery
and Biomedical Engineering Unit
McGill University

Results from a number of experiments suggest that sensations of muscle force are derived from corollaries of centrally generated motor commands (Jones and Hunter, 1983; McCloskey, 1981). Most of these studies have examined the effect of changing the state of the agonist muscle (e.g., by partial curarization, fatigue, or tendon vibration) on the perception of force (Gandevia and McCloskey, 1977; Jones and Hunter, 1985; McCloskey et al., 1974). However, under normal physiological conditions co-contraction of the antagonist muscle is often observed (Hepp-Reymond and Wiesendanger, 1972; Lamarre et al., 1981; Marsden et al., 1979). Although there have been several reports of changes in the perceived magnitude of the force of contraction when the antagonist muscle is co-contracting (Gandevia et al., 1980; Jones & Hunter, 1985), the effect of co-contraction on the perceived intensity of forces exerted by a limb has not been systematically investigated. Co-contraction occurs most frequently under conditions in which the control of force is of critical importance, such as during prehensile grasping (Smith, 1981). In this situation it appears to stablize the wrist and to stiffen the carpal and metacarpophalangeal joints. Co-contraction has also been reported during tasks that require carefully graded muscular activity, such as visual-tracking movements (Marsden et al., 1979). It has been hypothesized that under these conditions co-contraction acts as a brake to smooth the movement.

The degree of co-contraction can be voluntarily controlled in some muscle groups, although there appears to be an upper limit to the magnitude of the forces that can be generated simultaneously in the agonist and antagonist muscles (Hunter et al., 1983). Figure 1 shows the results obtained from one subject who was able to vary the level of triceps activation while simultaneously contracting the biceps muscle. The isometric forces measured at the wrists are plotted against the surface electromyogram (EMG) recorded from the biceps muscle. Four different levels of co-contraction were maintained by the subject, while he made ramp-force contractions which went from rest to maximum force. The progression of curves from right to left illustrates the dramatic effect that increasing the level of activation of the antagonist triceps muscle can have on the force-biceps EMG relation. When the forces exerted by the biceps and triceps muscles are equal the net force at the wrist is zero, even though both the biceps and triceps muscles are strongly activated. The line parallel to the axis of ordinates shows these data. These results indicate

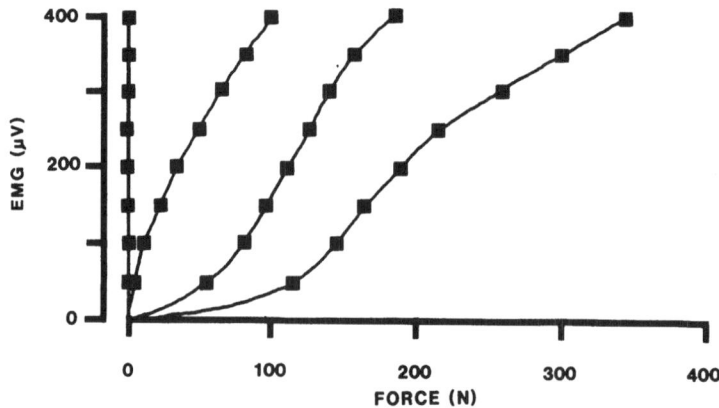

Fig. 1. The relation between the biceps EMG and the forces measured at the
wrist at four different levels of triceps co-contraction in one
subject.

that the shape of the force-EMG relation is highly dependent on the level
of antagonist activation.

These findings provided the basis for studying the effects of co-
contraction on the perception of force. In the present experiment a con-
tralateral-limb-matching procedure was used to assess how co-contraction of
the antagonist triceps muscle affected the perceived magnitude of forces
generated by the elbow flexors and extensors. Subjects were seated in an
experimental rig, and were strapped into the seat in order to minimize
movements of the trunk. The arms were spaced approximately 300 mm apart,
and the angle between the upper arm and the forearm was 90 degrees. EMGs
were recorded from the skin surface overlying the biceps and triceps
(lateral head) muscles of both arms. The isometric forces produced at the
wrists were measured by two strain gage force transducers and were recorded
on-line by a computer. The co-contraction levels for the biceps and triceps muscles were calculated from the EMGs measured during maximum voluntary contractions. Five EMG levels were used ranging in 10% increments
from 0% to 40% of the maximum EMG of each muscle. This gave a total of 25
trials. A visual target on an oscilloscope positioned in front of the
subject signalled the required degree of co-contraction. The amplified,
band-pass filtered (10 to 500 Hz), rectified, and then low-pass filtered
EMGs of the right biceps and triceps muscles were fed back to the subjects
as coordinates on the X-Y axes of the oscilloscope. Subjects were given 4
seconds to generate the target level of co-contraction. While maintaining
this reference contraction, they produced a perceptually equivalent force
with their left (matching) arm. These matching forces provided an estimate
of the perceived intensity of the reference arm contraction. The force and
EMG data were analyzed by calculating the mean force and EMG for both arms
during the last 1 second of each matching contraction.

The relation between the forces generated by the right, reference arm
and the matching forces is shown for a typical subject in Figure 2. The
line of equality in this figure indicates the values at which the reference
and matching forces are equal. Forces generated under conditions in which
there was no antagonist co-contraction were reasonably accurately matched
by the contralateral muscle group. However, when the triceps and biceps
muscles of the reference arm were co-contracting, the matching forces
exerted were in the direction of the more strongly activated muscle. That
is, the matching forces were flexion forces if the biceps was more active

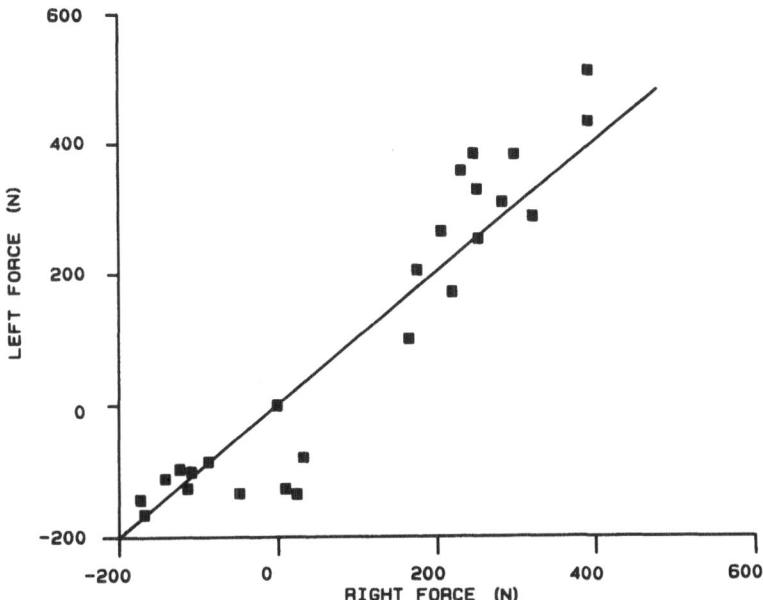

Fig. 2. The relation between the reference forces exerted by the right arm
and the matching forces produced by the left arm for a typical
subject. Negative forces represent forces generated predominantly
by the triceps muscles. The line of equality is shown.

than the triceps, and extension forces when the triceps was the more active
muscle. However, when matching the forces in the two limbs, subjects did
not consistently co-contract the muscles in the matching limb, even when
the two reference limb muscles were exerting quite high forces. The difference in the patterns of anonist-antagonist activation in the two limbs
is shown for one subject in Figure 3. Despite this difference in the level
of co-contraction in the two limbs, the matching forces can be predicted
reasonably well from the EMGs of the biceps and triceps muscles of the
reference arm. The variance accounted for by a multiple linear regression
using these two variables is 84%.

Co-contraction had a marked effect on the perceived magnitude of the
reference forces, however, this effect was not simply an additive one. The
perceived amplitude of forces produced by co-contracting the biceps and
triceps muscles at 20% of their respective maximum EMGs, was substantially
different from that produced when the biceps was at 30% and the triceps was
at 10%.

In summary, these results indicate that co-contraction does influence
the perception of force generated by a limb. However, there does not
appear to be a simple additive relation between the individual forces
generated by the agonist and antagonist muscles and the perceived intensity
of the overall contraction. Nevertheless, the matching forces can be
predicted from the EMGs of the reference-arm muscle group. It has been
suggested that the sense of heaviness is linked directly to the degree of
activation of the agonist muscle, and that the central nervous system does
not subtract or otherwise directly allow for activity in an antagonist
muscle (Marsden et al., 1979). However, these findings suggest that the
perception of force is derived not only from the efferent input to the
agonist muscle, but also from the input to other muscle groups involved in
the motor task.

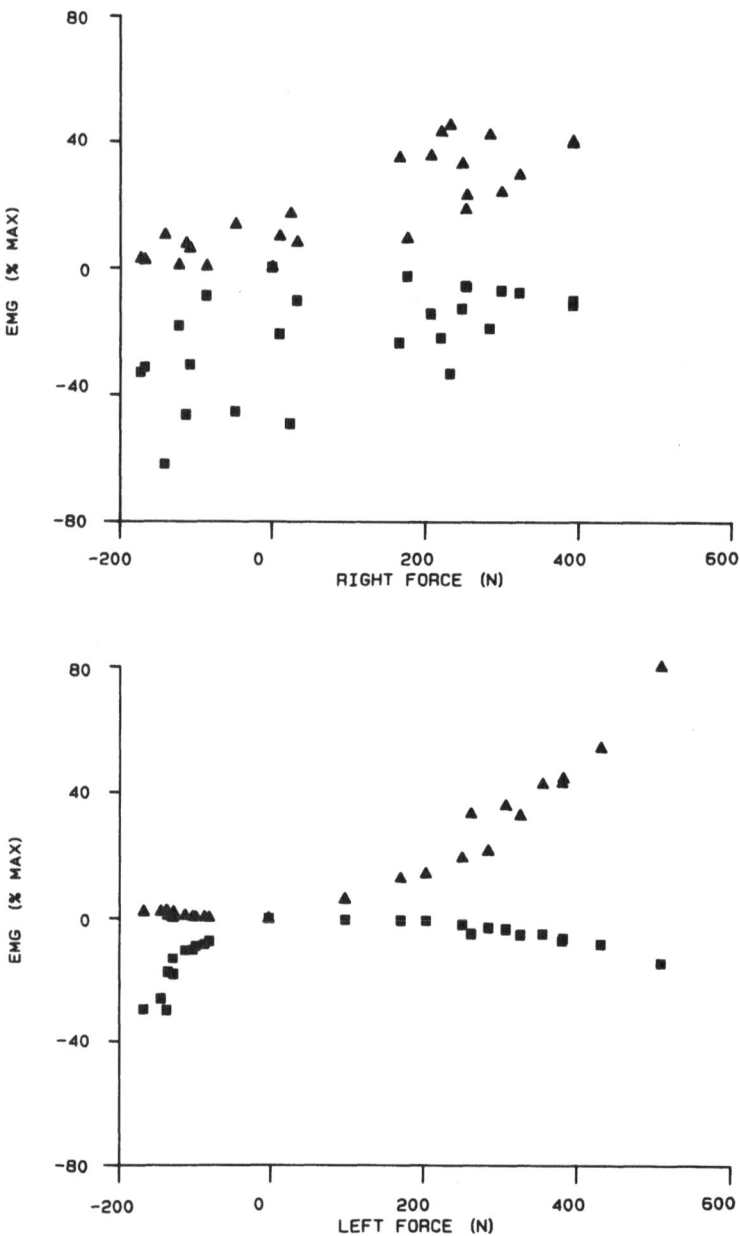

Fig. 3. The surface EMGs recorded from the biceps (triangles) and triceps
(squares) muscles during contractions generated by the reference
arm (upper plot) and matching arm (lower plot). Negative EMGs and
forces represent EMGs and forces recorded from the triceps muscle.

REFERENCES

Gandevia, S. C., and McCloskey, D. I., 1977, Changes in motor commands as
      shown by changes in perceived heaviness, during partial curarization
      and peripheral anaesthesia in man, J.Physiol., 272:673.
Gandevia, S. C., McCloskey, D. I., and Potter, E. K., 1980, Alterations in
      perceived heaviness during digital anaesthesia, J.Physiol., 306:365.

Hepp-Reymond, M. -C., and Wiesendanger, M., 1972, Unilateral pyramidotomy in monkeys: effect on force and speed of a conditioned precision grip, Brain Res., 36:117.

Hunter, I. W., Kearney, R. E., and Weiss, P. L., 1983, Variation of ankle stiffness with co-contraction, Soc.Neurosci.Abstr., 9:1226.

Jones, L. A., and Hunter, I. W., 1983, Effect of fatigue on force sensation, Exp.Neurol., 81:640.

Jones, L. A., and Hunter, I. W., 1985, Effect of muscle tendon vibration on the perception of force, Exp.Neurol., 87:35.

Lamarre, Y., Spidalieri, G., and Lund, J. P., 1981, Patterns of muscular and motor cortical activity during a simple arm movement in the monkey, Can.J.Physiol.Pharmacol., 59:748.

Marsden, C. D., Rothwell, J. C., and Traub, M. M., 1979, Effect of thumb anaesthesia on weight perception, muscle activity and the stretch reflex in man, J.Physiol., 294:303.

McCloskey, D. I., 1981, Corollary discharges: motor commands and perception, in: "Handbook of Physiology, The Nervous System," Vol.II, V. B. Brooks, ed., American Physiological Society, Bethesda.

McCloskey, D. I., Ebeling, P., and Goodwin, G. M., 1974, Estimation of weights and tensions and apparent involvement of a "sense of effort", Exp.Neurol., 42:220.

Smith, A. M., 1981, The coactivation of antagonist muscles, Can.J.Physiol. Pharmacol., 59:733.

INITIATION OF ELECTROMYOGRAPHIC ACTIVITY

IN FAST FORWARD ARM ELEVATION

P. Gatev, G. N. Gantchev, R. Koedjikova, and B. Dimitrov

Department of Motor Control, Institute of Physiology
Bulgarian Academy of Sciences
Sofia, Bulgaria

This study dealt with the temporal organization of the recruitment of the muscles involved in the fast forward arm elevation. We aimed to measure their electromyographic (EMG) onsets according to the EMG onset of the anterior deltoid (AD), a prime mover of the humerus flexion and to obtain data about the temporal organization of the final command to the muscles contributing to this complex ballistic multijoint movement at different body positions and types of arm loading.

Forward arm elevation to the horizontal includes at the shoulder joint; flexion of the humerus, slight outward rotation, possibly abduction if scapula is laterally tilted; at the shoulder girdle: slight upward rotation of the scapula, abduction and lateral tilt, unless inhibited (Inman et al., 1944, Basmajian, 1969, Wells, 1971). Thirteen muscles were investigated suitable for surface EMG recording. The AD and pectoralis major (clavicular portion) (PMc) muscles are the prime movers of the flexion at the shoulder joint and the long head of brachial biceps (BB1) is their assistant. Four parts of the trapezius muscle (TR) act as stabilizers of the scapula. In addition the second and fourth part of TR are movers of upward rotation of the scapula, acting as a force couple, and the third part of the TR is the key of lateral tilt as an antagonist of this movement. The infraspinatus and teres minor muscles (IS+TMi) are movers of outward rotation of the humerus with the posterior deltoid (PD) as their assistant. These muscles also neutralize the inward rotation of the humerus caused by AD. Besides, the horizontally running fibers of PD stabilize the shoulder joint. We should consider also that this muscle is an assistant mover of extension of the humerus. In the case of abduction of the humerus the middle deltoid muscle (MD) is the prime mover with the BB1 as an assistant. The sternal portion of the major pectoral (PMs) was found to be active in forward arm elevation too. This muscle is a prime mover of extension and adduction, stabilizer of the shoulder joint as a possible neutralizer of an excessive abduction. The external oblique abdominal muscles, sinister (OES) and dexter (OED), are stabilizers of the ribs especially in forceful movements at the shoulder joint. These thirteen muscles are the major part of the muscles involved in the fast forward arm elevation.

Five healthy men were investigated, without problems of articular and muscular origin. Four experimental series were made. In two of them the arm was unloaded, freely hanging downwards. In the first series the subject was easy standing and in the second one he was sitting in a chair with the back vertically supported. In the other two parallel series the subject was easy standing and the arm was loaded by a load of two kg. In the first one the load was in the hand and in the second one the same load was hanging in equilibrium on nonelastic flexible connections parallel to the body, and the load was handgripped exactly at the fist level before the movement. The subject was instructed after the preparatory and execution commands to elevate as fast as possible the right arm to the horizontal, keeping the elbow straight. Bipolar surface electrodes with interpole distance of 10 mm were placed over the skin above the muscle under study as far as possible from other muscles contributing to that movement. The electrodes were at one and the same place during the four series. A four-channel electromyograph Medicor with frequency band from 50 to 5000 Hz was used. Recruitment time of each muscle was measured from the first sign of EMG activity in the AD (taken for zero) to the first sign of EMG activity of the muscle under study directly from the screen of a six-channel display with residual luminiscence, with an error of measurement not exceeding 1 ms. The EMG onset was calculated as a mean of 15 trials and was given with 95% confidence limits. In an additional series the time to the rise in tension was measured by an attempt to movement at the same conditions of the experiment. No matter the arm was loaded or not, all muscles before the movement were silent. Sometimes a low grade postural activity in the TR appeared, but it vanished when the subject was asked to relax.

The mean time of the whole command to the muscles was from 51 ms in sitting position to 61 ms in the load hanging series (range from 36 to 84 ms). There was a considerable amount of individual variation of both the recruitment order of the muscles and the recruitment time of each muscle. This was also the case with the time from EMG onset of AD to the rise in tension (range from 19 to 48 ms). Nevertheless, only few of the muscles, if any, started significantly (p<0.05, two-tailed Student's test) after the rise in tension. Few of the muscles changed significantly their EMG onsets to the left or to the right when the subject was sitting, compared with the series standing, resulting in an insignificant shift of the mean time of the whole command (Figure 1). When the arm was loaded and the load was in the hand many muscles changed their EMG onsets significantly, mainly to the right and some muscles to the left (Figure 2), causing a significant shift of the mean time of the command to the right by an average of 10 ms. In the series load hanging few of the muscles changed their EMG onsets compared with the load in the hand series. There was no significant shift of the mean time of the whole command, but just a slight tendency to the left in few of the subjects, and the chronodispersion of the EMG onsets was a little bit higher (Figure 3). Figure 4 shows the start time positions of those of the muscles of all subjects, which EMG onsets differed significantly from the EMG onset of AD. Almost all muscles from the total number of 60 differed from AD, when the arm was loaded, and their number appeared to be smaller when the arm was unloaded. Secondly, there was no difference in the number of these muscles, comparing on one hand the standing and sitting series, and on the other hand the load in hand and load hanging series. Thirdly, the chronodispersion was slightly higher when the load was handing, compared with the load in hand series. We have calculated also the number of muscles with EMG onsets significantly different from the EMG onset of AD by one SD. This number was diminished by factor of two, when the arm was loaded, and by factor of four or five when the arm was unloaded.

The main result in this work is that arm loading caused significant shifts of EMG onsets of many of the muscles involved in fast forward arm elevation according to the EMG onset of AD mainly to the right and, as a consequence of that, a delay of the mean time of the command was observed. The delay was mainly due to the TR, PD, ISP+TMi, OED, OES. To reveal the

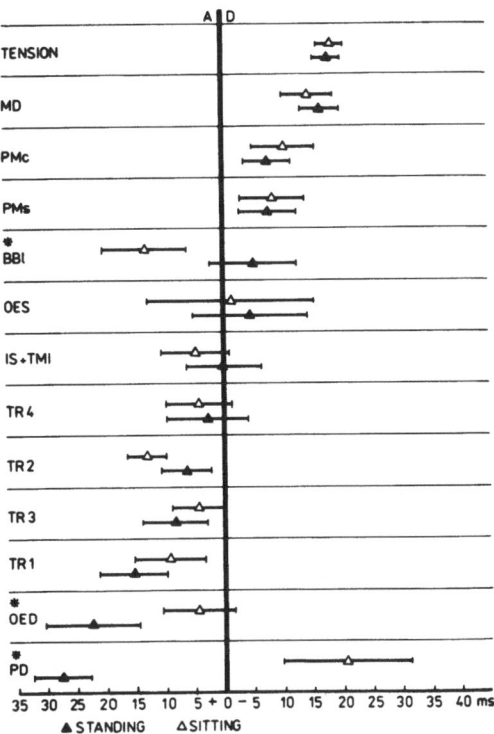

Fig. 1. Recruitment order of the muscles and time to the rise in tension
(mean with 95% confidence limits) of one of the subjects in the
series standing and sitting. The arrangement is according to the
EMG onsets in the series standing. *significant difference
(p<0.05, two-tailed Student's test) between the means of EMG
onsets of the muscle in the two series.

common feature of these muscles it is important to consider the fine inter-
play between all the muscles involved. They mutually neutralize their
functions not required at the moment, stabilize the joints and move the
load. There are many ways to perform these functions giving the reasons
for the great amount of individual variability. Only TR3, being an antagonist of the lateral tilt, showed a steady strategy. Other parts of TR
served to put the glenoidal fossa in the most favorable position to the
head of humerus. Nevertheless, by moving the origin of AD more medially
they acted like antagonists. Similar antagonistic functions might be
suggested for the OED and OES, which stabilize the ribs and play an antagonistic role with respect to the pectoralis minor and serratus anterior
muscles (not investigated), prime movers of lateral tilt of the scapula.
The delay of all these muscles with antagonistic functions will give an
advantage to the prime movers of flexion to move the load against inertia.
The early antagonist inhibition (Hufschmidt and Hufschmidt, 1958) may also
play role in that ballistic multijoint movement. The short duration of the
final command to the muscles and its time position, prevailingly before the
rise in tension, indicated its central programming. The suppression of
antagonists' motoneurons is most likely via Ia inhibitory interneurones, on
which converge influences from Ia afferents and corticomotoneuronal cells
(Jankowska et al., 1975, Kasser and Cheney, 1985). Reciprocal Ia inhibition during voluntary movements in man was found to increase with the
increase of contraction (Shindo et al., 1984). If we assume the speed of
movement and especially the early part of acceleration curve to be the main
programming variable (Bouisset and Lestienne, 1974), loading will be an

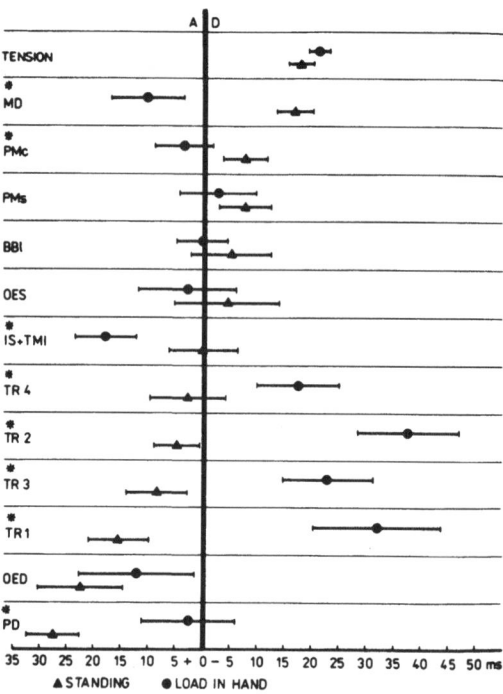

Fig. 2. Recruitment order of the muscles and time to the rise in tension of the same subject in the series standing and load in hand. The arrangement of EMG onsets is the same as on the Figure 1.

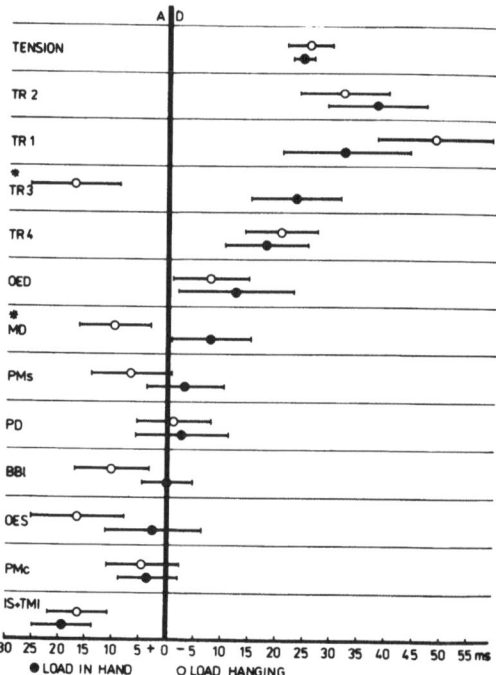

Fig. 3. Recruitment order of the muscles and the time to the rise in tension of the same subject in the series load in hand and load hanging. Note that arrangement is according to the sequence of the EMG onsets in the series load in hand.

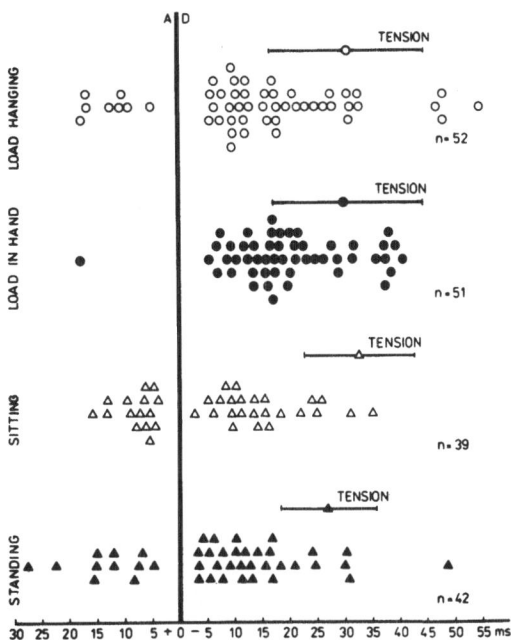

Fig. 4. Start time positions of those of all sixty muscles of five
subjects which mean of the EMG onset differed significantly
(p<0.05, Student's two-tailed test) from the EMG onset of AD in
the four series. Note that the time to the rise in tension is
given with mean ± SD for all subjects.

important limitation factor of fastest velocity and acceleration in our
case. The lack of some afferent information when the load is handing may
explain partly the slight tendency of the shift of the mean time of the
command to the left and its slightly higher chronodispersion, because, as
shown by Rudomin et al., 1974, excitability of Ia afferents' terminals may
be depressed severely under deep anesthesia. The change of the habitual
shoulder posture also may be taken into consideration.

REFERENCES

Basmajian, J. V., 1962, "Muscles Alive: Their Functions Revealed by
    Electromyography," Williams and Wilkins Co., Baltimore.
Bouisset, S., and Lestienne, F., 1974, The organization of a simple
    voluntary movement as analyzed from its kinematic properties, Brain
    Res., 71:451.
Hufschmidt, H. J., and Hufschmidt, A., 1954, Antagonist inhibition as the
    earliest sign of sensory-motor reaction, Nature, 174N.4430:607.
Inman, V. T., Saunders, J. R., and Abbott, L. C., 1944, Observations on the
    function of the shoulder joint, J.Bone Joint Surgery, 26:1.
Jankowska, E., Rudel, Y., and Tanaka, R., 1976, Disynaptic inhibition of
    spinal motoneurons from the motor cortex in the monkey, J.Physiol.,
    258:467.
Kasser, R. J., and Cheney, P. D., 1985, Characteristics of corticomoto-
    neuronal postspike facilitation and reciprocal suppression of EMG
    activity in the monkey, J.Neurophysiol., 53:959.
Rudomin, P., Nunez, R., Madrid, J., and Burke, R. E., 1974, Primary
    afferent hyperpolarization and presynaptic facilitation of Ia

afferent terminals induced by large cutaneous fibers, J.Neurophysiol., 37:413.

Shindo, M., Horayama, H., Kando, K., Ynagisono, M., and Tanaka, R., 1984, Changes in reciprocal Ia inhibition during voluntary contraction in man, Exp.Brain Res., 53:400.

Wells, K. F., 1971, "Kynesiology. The Scientific Basis of Human Motion," W. B. Saunders Co., Phyladelphia.

SECTION IV
POSTURE CONTROL

BULBAR RETICULAR UNIT ACTIVITY RELATING

TO POSTURE AND SKILLED FORELIMB MOVEMENT IN RATS

M. Šaling, J. Kundrát, and P. Duda

Institute of Normal and Pathological Physiology
Slovak Academy of Sciences
Bratislava, Czechoslovakia

Activity change of reticular neurons was observed in relation to single movements of head, neck, forelimb and facial muscles in unrestrained cats (Siegel and McGinty, 1977; Siegel, 1979). Congruent results were reported in the rat (Vertes, 1979). However, the relation of these reticular activity to single parts of movement is not elucidated. In the preceding work we observed depression of reticular unit activity connected with the execution of the forelimb movement and not with the preparatory phase (Šaling et al., 1985). The observed changes can be related to the forelimb movement itself or to the postural adjustments, accompanying this movement, or maybe to somesthetic feedback from the periphery. In the present paper we have therefore analyzed the relation of reticular unit activity to the postural changes or to the forelimb movement itself. The given problem was studied by means of the modified model of the "handedness of rat".

Ten male rats (Drucray strain) were trained to reach small pellets from horizontal tubes (inner diameter 11 mm) placed at two different levels (Figure 1). The animal reached the pellets either in the sitting position (lower place tube Figure 1A), or in the upright position (higher placed tube Figure 1C). We supposed the forelimb movement to be the same in both situations, but the postural adjustment to be different. The forelimb extension was detected by a photoelectrical sensor. For the next test we chose a rising rat to compare postural changes connected with single motor actions. The interrupting of the light beam just in front of the higher placed tube indicated the end of the rise. For computer processing photo-detection of single tested situations was differentiated by the generation of rectangular pulses of a different amplitude (Figure 1). Animals, which consistently reached pellets in the feeder by the right or the left forepaw were used in electrophysiological experiments. The metal guiding tubes were implanted in the trained rats above the bulbar medial reticular formation (RF) in pentobarbital anesthesia (SPOFA 50 mg/kg i.p.).

After the recovery of the animals a miniature micromanipulator with a glass micropipette was fixed to the guiding tube. Microelectrodes were filled with 4 M NaCl (tip resistance 2-10 MΩ). In the course of the experiment the microelectrodes were inserted through the intact dura meter and the cerebellum into the RF. Unit activity was recorded during spontaneous reaching and rising. Amplified signals (gain 1000 x) were tape-recorded and displayed on an oscilloscope. Records of activity 400 ms

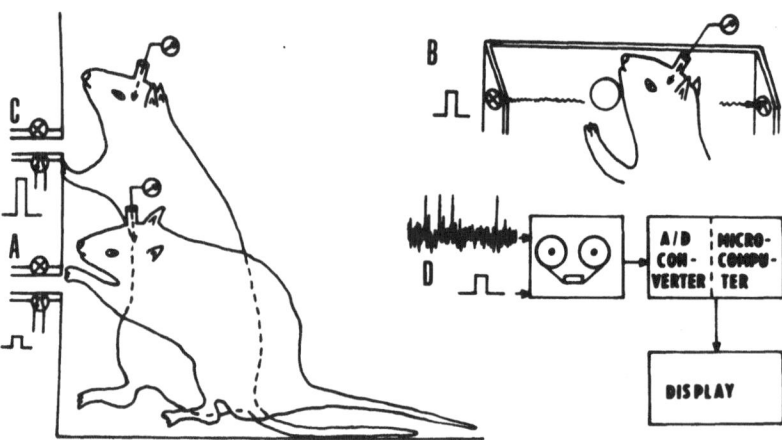

Fig. 1. Arrangement of experiment. (A) reaching of rat in the sitting position; (B) photodetection of the end of the rise; (C) reaching of rat in the upright position; (D) schema of processing of unit activity.

before and after the movement photodetection were evaluated by micro-computer. Spikes were automatically detected by the recognition computer program using amplitude, slope and duration parameters. Peri-event histograms were constructed from the detected spikes (bin = 16 ms).

We evaluated 20 reticular neurons, which satisfied the conditions of spike detection. Reticular neurons were recorded in the bulbar RF. We observed the periods of the increase or the depression of reticular unit activity in relation to the tested motor situation. The different behavior of unit activity relating to single tested situations was most frequent. In Figure 2 the reticular unit with different reaction in single motor action is documented. An increase of the reticular unit activity during reaching in the sitting position is presented in the raster of the individual trials. The peri-reach histogram has clearly documented the observed increase of unit activity, which appeared about 200 ms before the movement detection and lasted about 250 ms (Figure 2A). The activity peak of the increase is just before the movement detection. On the other hand during the reaching in the upright posture the same reticular neuron did not change its activity, as evident from the peri-reach histogram (Figure 2B). An activity depression of this reticular neuron was found in the rising rat (Figure 2B). The depression of activity started 200 ms before the movement detection and lasted 300 ms, culminating approximately at the onset of the movement. Other typical responses of neurons consisted in the facilitation or the depression of activity in one tested situation. In the other tested situations the reticular neuron did not change its activity. In two reticular neurons we found in both situations the same responses during the reaching. In one case there was a phasic excitation of 100 ms before the photodetection of movement and was followed by the inhibitory response. In the second neuron we observed a depression of activity just before the reach onset.

From the different reactions of reticular neurons in the single motor actions we can conclude that these reactions were related to postural changes. This is in agreement with the observation that the stimulation of the motor cortex after the pyramidal tract section is still effective in producing the postural adjustments (Nieoullon and Gahery, 1978). These facts support the hypothesis that the basic network for postural adjustments is located at the bulbospinal level (Massion and Gahery, 1979).

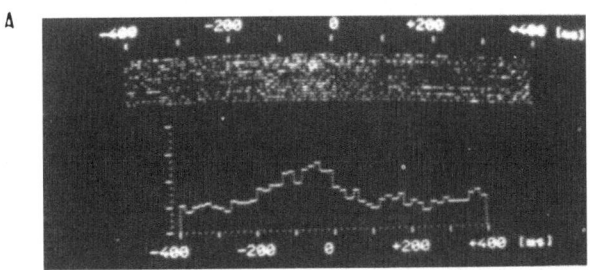

NUMBER OF REPEATING = 15
NUMBER OF SPIKES   = 931

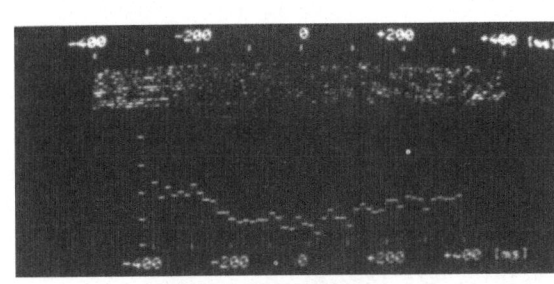

NUMBER OF REPEATING = 13
NUMBER OF SPIKES   = 879

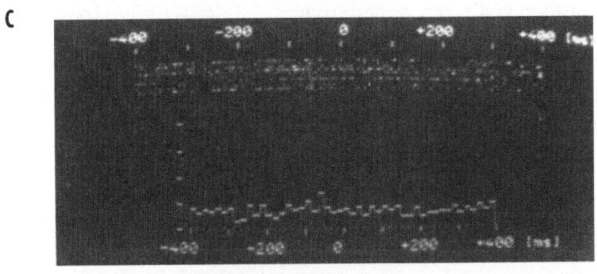

NUMBER OF REPEATING = 10
NUMBER OF SPIKES   = 444

Fig. 2. Unit activity changes of the same reticular neuron in the tested
         situations. (A) reaching in the sitting position; (B) the rise of
         rat; (C) reaching in the upright position. In the upper parts the
         raster of individual trials, in the lower parts the peri-event
         histograms (bin = 16 ms). Each division of vertical scale means
         two.

Reticular formation forms probably the main part of the network. The
pathways of medial reticular formation in cat establish connection preferentially with motoneurons of neck and back muscles (Wilson and Yoshida,
1969; Peterson, 1979). Only in two cases we observed the same activity
changes in both situations of reaching. These changes are probably related
to the forelimb movement itself. With regard to their timing they were
connected with the execution of the forelimb movement.

The present data suggest, that RF is able to participate in the fine
control of postural adjustment. The reticular participation in postural
control has a specific character. In this context it is relevant to
mention that the discharge activity of reticular neurons was directionally
related to head movements (Siegel, 1979) and in the course of stepping the
activity of reticulospinal neurons occurs with the swing phase of the step
(Orlovskii, 1970).

REFERENCES

Massion, J., and Gahery, Y., 1979, Diagonal stance in quadrupeds: a postural support for movement, in: "Reflex Control of Posture and Movement, Prog. in Brain Res.", R. Granit and O. Pompeiano, eds., vol. 50, Elsevier, Amsterdam.

Nieoullon, A., and Gahery, Y., 1978, Influence of pyramidotomy on limb flexion movements induced by cortical stimulation and on associated postural adjustment in the cat, Brain Res., 155:39-52.

Orlovskii, G. N., 1970, Work of the reticulo-spinal neurons during locomotion, Biophysics, 15:728-737 (in Russian).

Peterson, B. W., 1979, Reticulospinal projections to spinal motor nuclei, Ann.Rev.Physiol., 41:127-140.

Siegel, J. M., 1979, Behavioral relations of medullary reticular formation cells, Exp.Neurol., 65:696-716.

Siegel, J. M., and McGinty, D. J., 1977, Pontinne reticular formation neurons: relationship of discharge to motor activity, Science, 196:678-680.

Šaling, M., Pavlásek, J., Kundrát, J., and Duda, P., 1985, Activity changes in nucleus reticularis gigantocellularis in relation to skilled forelimb movement in rats, Brain Res., 331:137-141.

Vertes, R. P., 1979, Brain stem gigantocellularis neurons: patterns of activity during behavior and sleep in the freely moving rat, J.Neurophysiol., 42:214-228.

Wilson, V. J., and Yoshida, M., 1969, Comparison of effects of stimulation of Deiter's nucleus and medial longitudinal fasciculus on neck, forelimb and hindlimb motoneurons, J.Neurophysiol., 32:743-758.

PUTATIVE NEUROPHYSIOLOGICAL AND NEUROCHEMICAL MECHANISMS

UNDERLYING STRIATAL CONTROL OF POSTURAL ADJUSTMENT IN DOGS

K. B. Shapovalova and I. V. Yakunin

Laboratory and Physiology of Higher Nervous Activity
I. P. Pavlov Institute of Physiology Academy of Sciences
of the USSR, Leningrad, USSR

Though there are findings to indicate that striatum is probably involved in posture regulation (Martin, 1967; Villablanca et al., 1976; Johnels and Steg, 1980), no temporal analysis of the components of posture adjustment has been attempted so far. Neither has been done on the role of the striatal transmitters and, first of all, on the involvement of dopaminergic and cholinergic striatal system in the control of components of postural adjustment preceding voluntary movement.

Components of conditioned postural adjustment (Shapovalova et al., 1984) have been analysed (Figure 1) in chronic experiments on the model of instrumental defensive reaction connected with a certain posture maintenance (Petropavlovsky, 1934). Experiments were performed under the influence of different factors both on intact dogs and dogs with a different degree of caudate pathology. These factors are: electrical stimulation of the head of the caudate nucleus (HCN) in the right or left hemispheres by the implanted bipolar electrodes; systemic injections of L-Dopa (a dopamine agonist) and of haloperidole, blocking dopamine receptors; dopamine and carbocholine injection through the microcannulae into the HCN and into the "limbic" striatum structure - nucleus accumbens (NAC).

Preliminary low frequency stimulation of HCN (16 v, 2 Hz, 0.5 ms) switched on for 10 s before the onset of the conditioned signal (metronome, 130/min) significantly increased the duration of the main component of the postural adjustment (L_3), i.e., the time interval during which the weight of the working limb is unloaded and redistributed over the supporting limbs (Figure 2). A similar effect was produced by a bilateral carbocholine injection (1.0 mkg) into HCN and NAC (Figure 3). At the same time, this component of postural adjustment did not change with different modulations of dopamine levels in the HCN and NAC.

However, the initial components of postural adjustment, and, first of all, the latency of the beginning of the posture changes (L_1) sharply increased during systemic haloperidole injections (Figure 2) and significantly decreased during systemic L-Dopa administration and after dopamine injections (3.0 mkg) into HCN and NAC (Figure 4). It was also shown that microinjections of dopamine into NAC both in intact dogs and dogs with caudate pathology significantly increased the amplitude of the voluntary response, but dopamine injections into HCN did not elicit such effects. On the contrary, bilateral carbocholine injections into NAC significantly

123

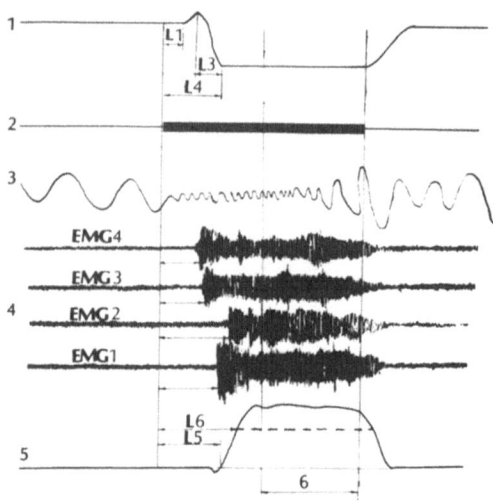

Fig. 1. Recording apparatus and processing of the data. (1) recording of pressure changes upon the tensoplatform by the working limb: L_1, latent period of the beginning of the posture adjustment; L_3, time interval of unloading the working limb, which corresponds to its weight shift upon the supporting limbs; L_4, latent period of the total posture adjustment. (2) the conditioned signal onset (metronome, 130/min). (3) respiration recording. (4) EMG records for the working (back, left) and for the supporting (back, right) limbs: EMG_1, latency of EMG-activity m.rectus femoris; EMG_2, latency of EMG-activity m.semitendinosus of the working limb; EMG_3, EMG_4, the same for the supporting limb. (5) the mechanogram of the working limb: L_5, latent period of the instrumental movement; L_6, latent period of the instrumental task solution (time necessary for the animal to hit a "safety zone"). (6) duration of the electrical current passed.

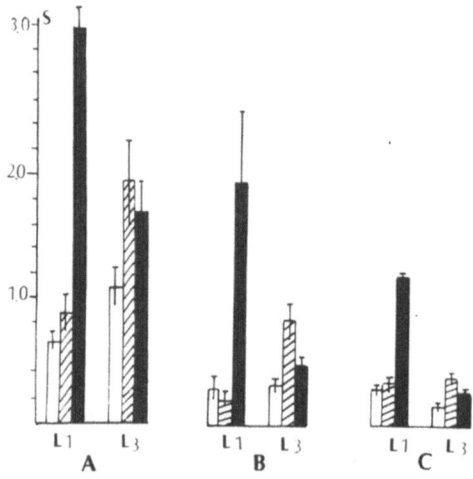

Fig. 2. Effects of the preliminary low-frequency stimulation of the HCN (hatched columns) and of the systemic haloperidole injections 0.1 mg/kg (filled black columns) upon the temporal characteristics (s) of the components of posture adjustment (L_1 and L_3) in three dogs (A,B,C). Empty white columns - background. Mean data (n=21).

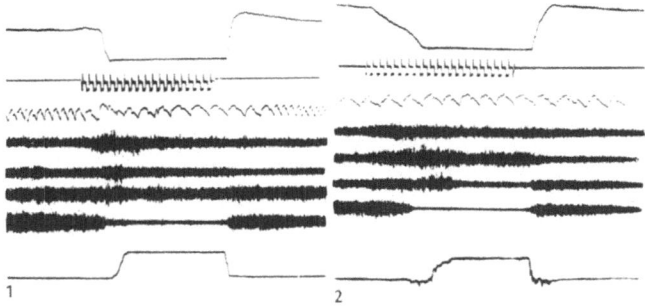

Fig. 3. Effects of bilateral carbocholine microinjections into the HCN
upon the posture adjustment. (1) before the injection; (2) at the
30 min after the microinjection. From top to bottom: recording of
the tensogram of the working limb, the onset of the conditioned
signal (metronome, 130/min), recording of respiration, EMG_4, EMG_3,
EMG_2, EMG_1, mechanogram of the instrumental movement.

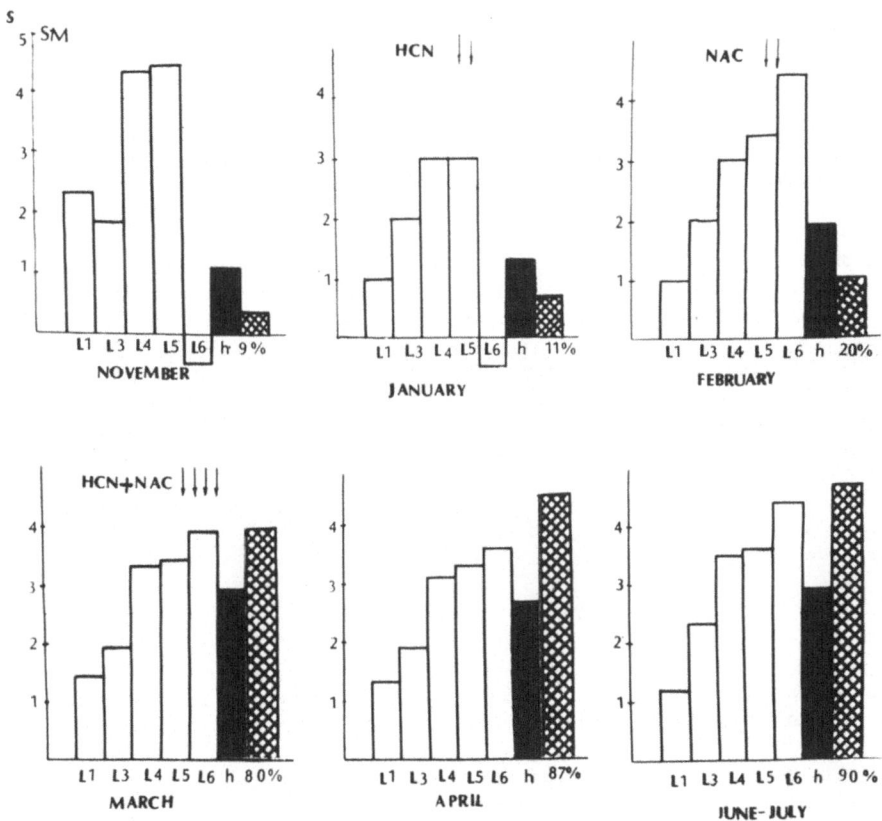

Fig. 4. Mean values (throughout a month) of the conditioned posture
adjustment components (L_1, L_3, L_4), the latent period of the
instrumental response (L_5), the latent period of the instrumental
task solution (L_6), s - white columns; the amplitude of the
instrumental response (h), sm - black columns, and percentage of
the correct instrumental responses - hatched columns. Before
(November) and after dopamine microinjections into dopaminergic
structures of the brain (January-July). The dog with a caudate
pathology.

decreased the amplitude of the voluntary movement in all animals. It should be noted that separate bilateral dopamine injections into HCN and into NAC elicit facilitatory effects only on the day of the injection and the day after it. Simultaneous bilateral dopamine microinjections into HCN and NAC, however elicit, prolonged effects especially in the dogs with a caudate pathology. In the latter case facilitatory effects persisted during four months (Figure 4).

Data obtained suggest that various components of the conditioned posture adjustment seem to be controlled by different striatal neurochemical mechanisms. Recent evidence allowed to formulate the idea (Groves, 1983) of two efferent systems of the neostriatum, differing in their morphological and neurochemical organization and in the effects they evoke on their major targets: globus pallidus and pars reticulata of the substantia nigra – inhibitory GABA-ergic influences (SI system) and activating P-ergic influences (SII system). Consequently the inhibitory effect of HCN stimulation may be associated with the disfunction of the SI system of the striatum and/or with the activation of cholinergic mechanism and as the result, with the direct involvement of SII system. In any case, either decreased dopamine-GABA-ergic effects and/or increased choline-P-ergic effects increase inhibitory pallidal and nigral influence upon the thalamic nuclei and midbrain motor structures (Kitai, 1981; Wise, 1984).

Clinical observations led to the conclusion that the endogenic neurotransmitters dopamine and acetylcholine are opposite in their action in the extrapyramidal system (Lehman and Langer, 1983). It was also suggested that the nigral dopamine-GABA-ergic/cholinergic balance is involved in the posture regulation (De Montis et al., 1979). Our studies provide direct evidence that the dopaminergic system of HCN is of critical value for the initiation of postural adjustment. Besides, the cholinergic system of the striatum is shown to be of great importance for the regulation of the main component of postural adjustment in dogs, i.e., for the unloading of the working limb due to the redistribution of weight upon the supporting limbs.

The observed postural changes elicited by dopamine and carbocholine microinjections into the NAC appeared unidirectional to those produced by microinjections of these drugs into HCN. Neuromorphological and neurochemical specificity of the NAC organization may explain the fact that its efferent influences activate dopaminergic mechanisms of the striatum (Mogenson et al., 1980; Shapovalova, 1985). It may be suggested, that these two structures are involved in the control of the posture interacting at the level of globus pallidus.

REFERENCES

De Montis, G. M., Olianas, M. C., Serra, G., Tagliamonte, A., and Scheel-Kruger, J., 1979, Evidence that a nigral GABA-ergic-cholinergic balance controls posture, Europ.J.Pharmacol., 53:181.

Groves, Ph. M., 1983, A theory of the functional organization of the neostriatum and neostriatal control of voluntary movement, Brain Res. Rev., 5:109.

Johnels, B., and Steg, G., 1980, The corpus striatum and the regulation of posture and locomotion, Neurosci.Lett., 19, Suupl. 5:339.

Kitai, S. T., 1981, Electrophysiology of corpus striatum and brain stem integrating systems, in: "Handbook of Physiology", J. M. Brookhart and V. B. Mountcastle, eds., Amer. Physiol. Soc., Bethesda (Md).

Lehmann, J., and Langer, S. Z., 1983, The striatal cholinergic interneuron: synaptic target of dopaminergic terminals?, Neuroscience, 10:1105.

Martin, J. P., 1967, "The Basal Ganglia and Posture", Pitman Med. Publ., London.

Mogenson, G. J., Johnes, D. L., and Yim, Ch. Y., 1980, From motivation to action: functional interface between the limbic system and the motor system, Progr.in Neurobiol., 14:69.

Petropavlovski, V. P., 1934, The method of conditional movement reflexes, Fiziol.Zh.im.I.M.Sechenova, 17:217 (in Russian).

Shapolvalova, K. B., 1985, Possible neurophysiological and neurochemical mechanisms of striatum involvement in the regulation of the voluntary movement, Fiziol.Zh.im.I.M.Sechenova, 71:537 (in Russian).

Shapovalova, K. B., Yakunin, I. V., and Boyko, M. I., 1984, Participation of dogs caudate nucleus head in the mechanisms of conditioned posture reorganization, Zh.Vyssh.Nervn.Deyat.im.I.P.Pavlova, 34:669 (in Russian).

Wise, S. P., 1984, Saccadic eye movement in response to drug action in the midbrain, Trends in Neurosci., 7:357.

ROLE OF THE VISUAL FEEDBACK FOR STABILIZATION OF VERTICAL

HUMAN POSTURE DURING INDUCED BODY OSCILLATIONS

G. N. Gantchev, P. Gatev, N. Tankov, N. Draganova*
S. Dunev*, and D. Popivanov

Institute of Physiology, Bulgarian Academy of Sciences
*Institute of Hygiene, Medical Academy, Sofia

The basic approach for studying the sensory control of posture activity and sensory interaction in this control is attenuation, deformation or interruption of the sensory inflow. Another approach for studying the posture control is to add supplementary information about body position and body oscillations via a sensory channel. Our studies have shown that the information for the spontaneous body sway provided by visual feedback (VFB) leads to stabilization of vertical human posture (Gantchev et al., 1979).

A recent report questioned the influence of the VFB upon the induced body oscillations. We have utilized the induced body oscillations as a model for studying postural control because of the advantages which it possesses (Gantchev, 1985): the body sway involves characteristic biomechanical changes; rhythmic changes in the biomechanics of posture with different frequency cause dynamic changes of the sensory inputs in different combinations; in those conditions various spinal and supraspinal mechanisms of postural control are involved including the mechanisms of volitional control.

METHODS

The method used for producing induced body oscillations of a standing subject was described previously (Dunev and Gantchev, 1972). The subject stood on a platform which could be rotated about an axis colinear with the axis of the ankle joint. Sinusoidal platform rotations with constant amplitude of 6° and frequency range 0.03, 0.01, 0.3, 0.5, 0.6, 0.7, 0.8 and 1 Hz were used in this study.

Stabilogram (SG) in anterio-posteior direction was recorded by means of tensometric transducer connected to the body at the level of gravity center (Dunev and Gantchev, 1972).

Goniogram (GG) of the ankle joint and surface EMG from soleus and tibialis muscles were recorded.

The information for body position and body oscillations was provided by visual feedback – 4 times amplified SG was displayed on the monitor at the level of the gaze of the experimental subject. The SG, GG and EMG were stored on a 4-channel tape recorder "Hewllet-Packard" for subsequent processing. Ten runs of SG, GG and rectified EMG were averaged by means of MING-23. Peak to peak amplitudes of averaged SG and GG were measured. Phase relationship between SG and GG were measured digitally. Integrated EMG (IEMG) for one cycle was recorded automatically.

Seven healthy subjects took part in the experiments. They were instructed to keep stable vertical posture in all experimental conditions: recording of SG for each frequency of platform rotations with and without VFB. The experimental sessions were randomly mixed. To avoid tiredness after one or two sessions subjects rested for enough time for recuperation.

RESULTS

In Figure 1 are presented the mean values for all subjects of the amplitude of induced sway at different platform rotations.

The data showed that the amplitude of induced oscillations was about 3 cm 0.03 Hz. If the body follows the displacement of the platform at constant angle of the ankle joint, the deviation at the level of gravity center should be about 10 cm. Therefore considerable compensation of the body sway induced by platform rotation occurred at lowest frequency of rotation.

The amplitude of the induced body oscillations decreased with increasing frequency of platform rotation. The decrease of the amplitude occurred up to 0.5 Hz. After this frequency of platform rotation no changes in the amplitude of the sway were observed. Similar changes of the amplitude of induced body oscillations related to the frequency of platform displacement were shown in our previous studies (Gantchev et al., 1972; Gantchev and Popov, 1973) and confirmed in the study of Walsh (1973) and Gurfinkel et al. (1976). Diner et al. (1982) found higher amplitude of body sway at low frequency of platform rotation - about 6-7 cm - as well as at the highest frequency. These differences were probably due to the dynamic component of SG recorded by force platform which was the case with the studies of Diner et al. (1982).

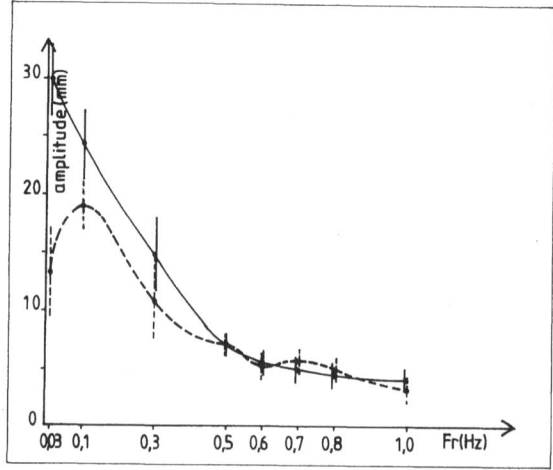

Fig. 1. Amplitudes of the induced body oscillations at different frequencies of platform rotations. (--------) with VFB; (————) without VFB.

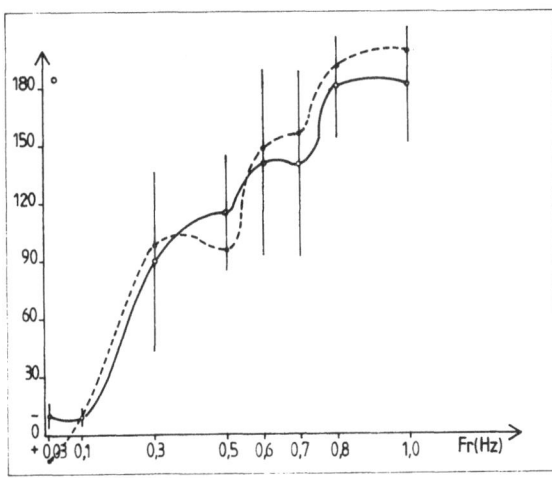

Fig. 2. The phase lead of the body oscillations (in angular degree) at
different frequencies of platform rotations. (————) in
forward and (--------) backward deviation of the body.

Figure 2 shows mean value for all subjects of phase shift at different
frequencies of platform rotation. It is seen that at low frequencies the
maximum of SG practically coincides with the maximum and minimum of the GG
– sometimes preceding or slightly delayed. At higher frequencies a phase
lead was observed – the higher the frequencies, the higher the phase lead.
At the highest frequency of 1 Hz a considerable phase lead was observed
which amounted to 180° and more on the average. That is the reason for
antiphase of the SG and GG being observed. In two subjects the phase lead
was more than 180°. These data are in agreement with the results of Diner
et al. (1982), who have found positive phase lead at lowest frequencies up
to 0.01 Hz and negative phase lead at higher frequencies.

The phase lead was about the same for body deviation forward and
backward.

IEMG of soleus and tibialis ant.msucles is presented in Figure 3.
The data showed increase of IEMG with increasing frequency of platform
rotation. IEMG at 0.03 and 0.01 Hz was very low. It is almost equal or
slightly higher to the IEMG of soleus muscle at easy standing. This was
shown in the records of the IEMG of soleus muscle of another 7 subjects.
The increase of IEMG of soleus and tibialis ant.muscles developed up to
0.5 Hz. Between 0.5-0.7 Hz there was a plateau and after that a steep
increase at 0.8-1.0 Hz.

In Figure 1 are presented also the mean values for the amplitude of
the induced body oscillations for all subjects with VFB. It is seen that
at slow oscillations of the body the stabilizing effect of VFB is well
expressed. This effect is valid up to 0.3 Hz frequency of the platform
rotation.

The data showed that the phase lead of the SG was smaller with VFB up
to 0.5 Hz, but the differences were not significant. The time course of
the IEMG at different frequencies was similar at the two experimental
conditions, but at 1.0 Hz the IEMG for soleus muscle was significantly
smaller with VFB.

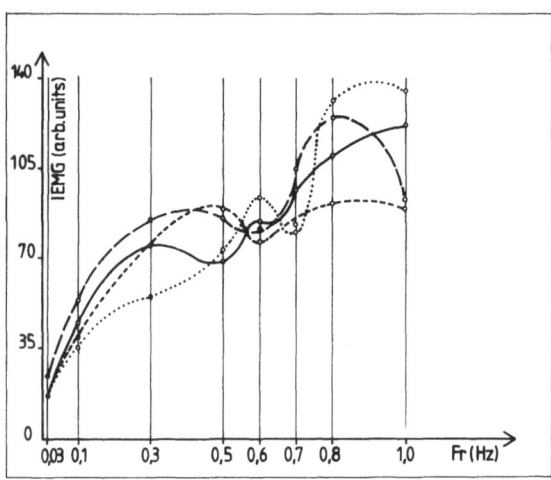

Fig. 3. Integrated EMG of soleus and tibialis ant. muscles at different
frequencies of platform rotations with VFB and without VFB.
(········) Sol. no VFB; (--------) Sol. VFB; (— — — —) Tib. VFB;
(————) Tib. no VFB.

DISCUSSION

The considerable compensation of the body sway in sagital plane at the
lowest frequency of the platform rotation is of interest. This compensation might be due to active forces, to muscle stiffness, to correction
via vestibular apparatus and proprioception. We believe that muscle
stiffness plays an important role for stabilizing vertical posture at the
lowest frequency. The absence of difference of IEMG at slow body sway and
easy standing is in support of this assumption. Studies of Nashner et al.
(1976) with rotational perturbation of ankle joint have shown that stabilization was achieved by inherent stiffness of the muscles. We suppose that
with the circumstances of our study the compensation of the body oscillations was assisted by the central regulation of muscular stiffness, and
by influences from muscle spindles as well (Allum and Mauritz, 1984).

The diminution of the amplitude of the oscillations while increasing
the frequency of platform movement was observed up to 0.5 Hz. Active
forces are added and together with passive forces and forces of inertia
take part in the maintenance of body stability. Studies of Gurfinkel
(1973) have shown that the acceleration increased strongly above 0.3-0.5 Hz
and is maximal around 1 Hz. Our data have shown that in fact the IEMG
increased considerably above 0.8 Hz. It is of interest to notice that in
the range of 0.5-0.7 Hz the changes of IEMG was comparably small.

When regularly stretching the muscles of the leg conditions arise for
the occurrence of stretch reflex as the stretching with greater velocities
is above threshold levels, and additionally, the threshold of the stretch
reflex decreases with muscle activation. In our study of regular body
oscillations an increase of soleus activity was observed in plantar flexion
but not in dorsiflexion when stretching of the muscle occurred. This was
shown in our previous studies (Gantchev and Draganova, 1976) and in the
studies of Gurfinkel et al. (1976). These results prove that stretch
reflex has no regulatory role upon vertical stance in the situation of
induced body oscillations.

The sensory systems participating in the regulation of vertical stance
are involved in different degree and combination among them, especially

with different frequency of platform movement. Passive elastic forces, vestibular apparatus and to a certain degree the visual system are dominating at very slow oscillations. The proprioceptive input, being under strong supraspinal control, dominates with increase of the oscillations. The role of the peripheral mechanisms increases too. This is obvious from the changes of the monosynaptic excitability during different phases of body oscillations tested by H-reflex. These changes closely correlate with the stretching and relaxation (i.e., activation) of the soleus muscle. The synthesis of information from vestibular apparatus and proprioreceptors is of interest, as it is expressed in different time intervals due to considerable phase delay of body movements compared to the platform rotations.

Differentation of the frequency domains of participation of the sensory systems in the control of the postural activity was specified by Nashner (1979) and later investigated concerning the visual system. According to Dichgangs and Brandt (1978) the visual system exerts its influence on body oscillations in the frequency domain between 0.1 and 1.0 Hz. The data of Walsh (1973) showed influence of the visual system in the frequency range 0.2-0.5 Hz. Recent studies of Diner et al. (1982) have shown that the influence of the visual system was expressed even at lower frequencies. Our study supports these data, i.e., the VFB of body oscillations stabilized body balance at low frequency domain down to 0.03 Hz. Regarding the upper frequency, it was found that there is no effect above 0.3 Hz. The stabilizing effect of the VFB could reach the limit of 0.6 Hz for the subjects well trained to perform the experimental task. This shows that the stabilizing effect of the visual system on upright posture could be improved by learning and that the restrictions in the control of the vertical body position are not due to the motor, but rather to the sensory part of the control system. This conclusion should be of important practical value for rehabilitation of the disrupted equilibrium.

REFERENCES

Allum, J. H. J., and Mauritz, K. H., 1984, Compensation for intrinsic stiffness by short-latency reflexes in human triceps surae muscles, J.Neurophysiology, 52:797.
Diner, H. C., Dishgangs, J., Bruzek, W., and Selinka, H., 1982, Stabilization of human posture during induced oscillations of the body, Exp. Brain Res., 45:126.
Dishgangs, J., and Brandt, T., 1978, Visual-vestibular interaction. Effects on self-motion perception and postural control, in: "Handbook of Sensory Physiology", P. Held and H. Liebowitz, eds., pp. 755, Springer, Berlin, Heidelberg, New York.
Dunev, S., and Gantchev, G. N., 1972, Une methode pour l'etude des oscillations due corps spontanees ou induites, Le Travail Humain, 35:267.
Gantchev, G. N., Dunev, S., and Draganova, N., 1972, On the problem of the induced body oscillations, Agressologie, 14B:51.
Gantchev, G. N., and Popov, V., 1973, Quantitative evaluation of induced body oscillations in man, Agressologie, 14C:91.
Gantchev, G. N., and Draganova, N., 1976, H-reflex changes in various phases of spontaneous and induced body oscillations, Agressologie, 17B:43.
Gantchev, G. N., Draganova, N., and Dunev, S., 1979, The role of the sensory feedback in the control of postural tonic activity, Agressologie, 20B:155.
Gurfinkel, E. V., 1973, Physical foundations of stabilography, Agressologie, 14C:9.
Gurfinkel, V. S., Lipshits, M. I., Mori, S., and Popov, K. E., 1976, Postural reactions to the controlled sinusoidal displacement of the supporting platform, Agressologie, 17B:71.

Nashner, L. M., 1976, Adapting reflexes controlling the human posture, Exp. Brain Res., 26:59.

Walsche, E. G., 1973, Standing man, slow rhythmic tilt, importance of vision, Agressologie, 14C:79.

AFFERENT CONTROL OF POSTURE AND GAIT

J. Quintern, W. Berger and V. Dietz

Department of Clinical Neurology and Neurophysiology
University of Freiburg, Freiburg i. Br.
West Germany

INTRODUCTION

Investigations of the complex movements involved in human posture and gait have been restricted to the description of the efferent arm of the movement, in the form of biomechanical data and muscle electromyographic (EMG) activity. The extent to which the latter, while being generated by a central program, was also influenced by spinal reflex systems became evident when fast movements were studied, such as running and jumping (Dietz et al., 1979; Dietz and Noth, 1978) or falling forward onto extended arms (Dietz et al., 1981). In addition, when unexpected displacements were induced during posture and gait (Berger et al., 1984), they evoked rapid appropriate and powerful EMG responses. The nature of these spinal reflex mechanisms, their afferent sources and their pathways, has remained a matter for debate. From experiments in the cat, many spinal reflex connections and interneuronal circuits involved in motor control are known (for review see Baldissera et al., 1981). Furthermore, there exists the possibility for selection of afferent information by presynaptic inhibition of afferent pathways to the spinal cord (Schmidt, 1971). However, little emerges from these experiments about the functional significance of different reflex pathways in the control of locomotion and it remains questionable if these spinal mechanisms can validly be transferred to the bipedal gait of man.

The aim of this Chapter will be to show some new aspects of the control of afferent information in human posture and gait and their significance in the compensation of unexpected displacements.

Inhibition of Monosynaptic Stretch Reflexes during Gait

For our investigations of the control of human posture and gait, the EMG of lower leg muscles was recorded using surface electrodes. Ankle joint movements were indicated by goniometers, while contact of the heel and ball of the foot was signalled by electrical contact switches fixed to the shoes (see Figure 1). The experiments were performed on a treadmill which allowed one to introduce fast acceleration impulses (capacity of the amplifier was 12750 W for 1 s) during posture and gait. The EMG was rectified and was transferred, together with the other data, to a computer system (Sirius) for averaging and further processing (for details see Berger et al., 1984).

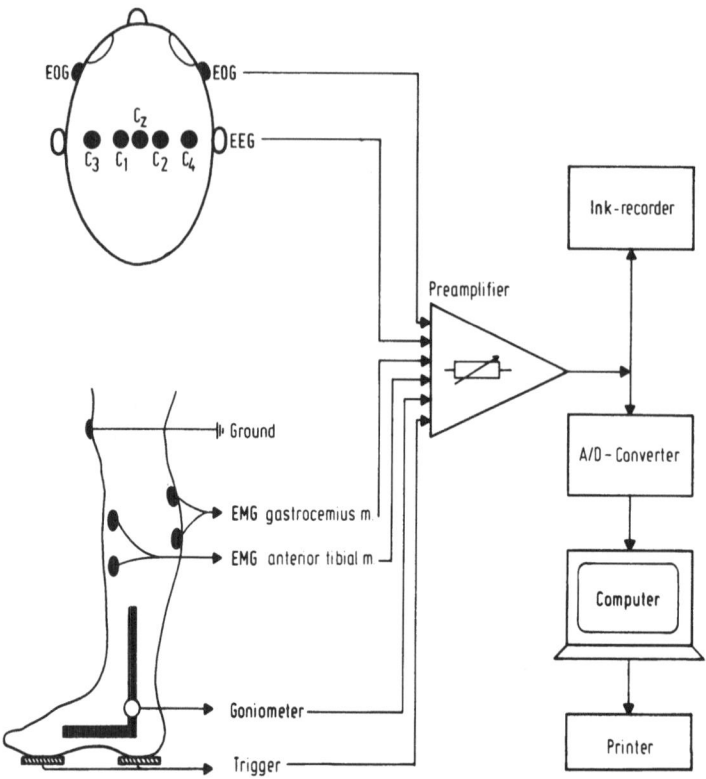

Fig. 1.   Schematic illustration of the parameters recorded and analyzed.

To investigate the relative contribution of different reflex systems
in the compensation of perturbations, three different modes of stretch were
applied to the triceps surae (Dietz et al., 1984): (1) when the foot of the
relaxed leg was quickly dorsiflexed, only a biphasic potential appeared,
with monosynaptic latency; (2) when, during posture, an acceleration
impulse was induced which displaced the legs in a posterior direction, the
triceps surae of both sides were stretched at a high velocity. In this
case, the small monosynaptic reflex response was followed by a strong
gastrocnemius EMG response (latency 70-75 ms); and (3) when the same impulse was applied at the beginning of the stance phase of gait, a monosynaptic stretch reflex response was lacking and only the strong longer
latency gastrocnemius (GM) response appeared. Despite the fact that the
GM was stretched at a high velocity (250-300 deg/s), monosynaptic stretch
reflex responses were never seen following these perturbations. This is
in accordance with the observed depression of the H-reflex during gait,
reported else where (Morin et al., 1982).

Our conclusion, that the strong, functionally essential, longer
latency GM response is not mediated by group I muscle proprioceptive
afferents is based on the observation that the response was preserved after
the group I afferents of the leg were blocked by ischemia (Berger et al.,
1984).

It is concluded from these experiments that the EMG responses may be
mediated predominantly by peripheral information from group II and group
III afferents, which modulate the basic motor pattern of spinal interneuronal circuits underlying the respective motor task. The absence of
effect of group I afferent input could be explained by presynaptic

inhibition of group I afferents during human gait, a mechanism demonstrated in cat experiments (Schmidt, 1971).

Suppression of Supraspinal Transmission from Group I Afferents during Gait

Projections from group I afferents to supraspinal motor centers are believed to play an important role in motor control (for review see Wiesendanger and Miles, 1982). To investigate the supraspinal transmission of group I afferents during human posture and gait, the electroencephalogram (EEG) was recorded over the precentral region (see Figure 1). The tibial nerve was stimulated at twice the motor threshold and the cerebral potentials (CP) evoked by this stimulus were analyzed (for further details see Dietz et al., 1986). Figure 2 shows the mean values of the CP evoked during posture and gait in 4 subjects. During gait the CP appeared with a longer latency (60 compared to 40 ms) and a smaller amplitude compared to those seen during posture, although care had been taken to hold the stimulus constant in both conditions (proved by recording the EMG over the abductor hallucis muscle). The assumption that these differences are really due to an inhibition of group I afferents was supported by the observation that after blockade of group I afferents by ischemia, the CP evoked by tibial nerve stimulation during posture were quite similar to those seen during gait (without ischemia; see Figure 2).

The same differences in latency and profile were seen when the CP were evoked by perturbations of posture and gait, with the exception that the CP evoked by these mechanical, quasi-natural, stimuli were 3 to 4 times larger in amplitude (Dietz et al., 1985; 1986). It is concluded that group I afferents are inhibited over their supraspinal pathway during gait and that

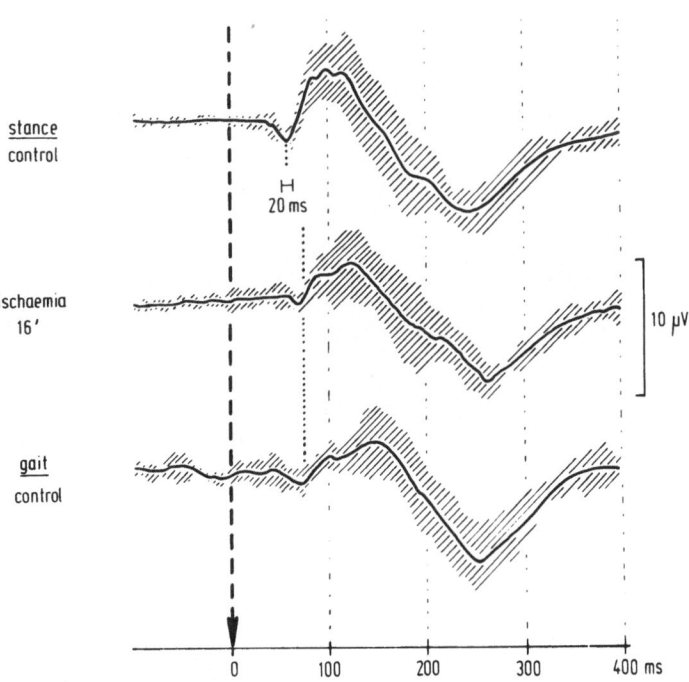

Fig. 2. C.p. (average of 40 to 100 stimuli) evoked by suprathreshold tibial nerve stimulation in three different conditions. From top to bottom: During stance; During stance after ischaemic nerve (group I afferents) blockade of the stimulated leg; During gait (normal condition). The mean values of 4 subjects are displayed.

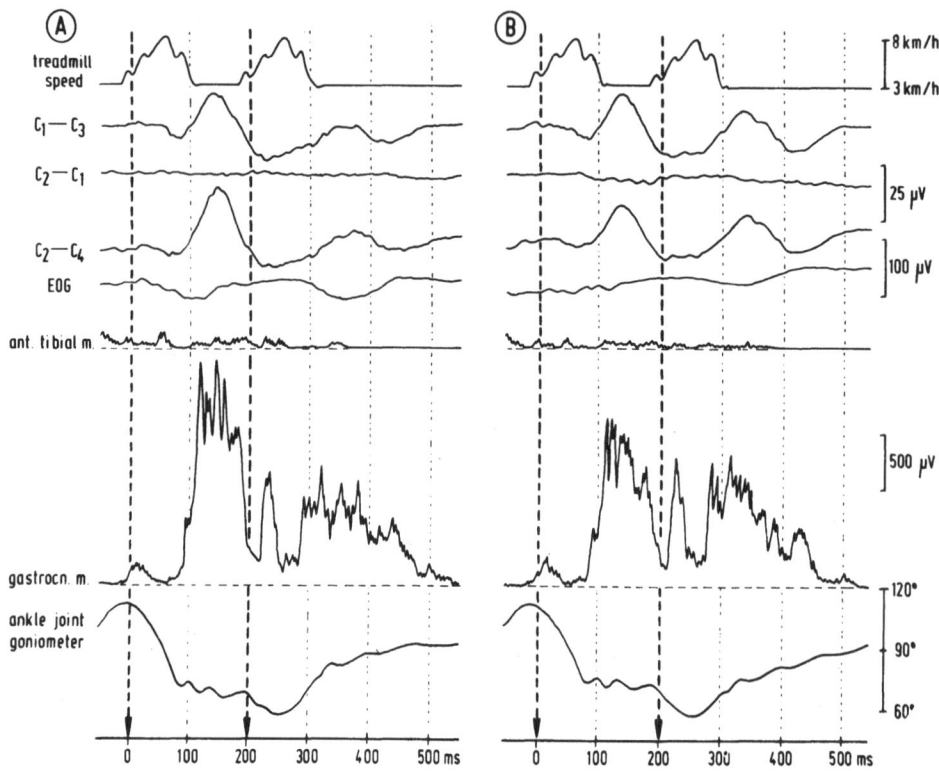

Fig. 3. C.p. (average of 30 trials) and e.m.g. responses (rectified and averaged, n=30) together with the ankle joint movements, evoked by randomly applied treadmill acceleration impulses at the beginning of the stance phase of gait. In (A) the subject was informed that the first perturbation impulse would be followed by a second one; in (B) a second impulse was induced unexpectedly.

the large CP amplitude in the latter task reflects a central processing of afferent input by supraspinal motor centers. This was shown to be a necessary preparation for a possible fall forwards induced by the perturbation impulses (Quintern et al., 1985).

In Figure 3 the CP evoked by gait perturbations are shown under two different conditions. In A the subject was informed beforehand that the first perturbation would be followed a short time later (200 ms) by a second one, while in B the second perturbation was induced unexpectedly. While the CP evoked by the first perturbation were about the same in A and B, the CP evoked by the second perturbation were larger when the second perturbation was induced unexpectedly (B). This observation supports the notion that psychological factors, such as predictability and practice, influence the amplitude of the CP evoked by a perturbation, while the compensatory EMG responses in the legs were only slightly affected by these factors (Quintern et al., 1985).

Figure 4 shows the distribution over the scalp of the CP evoked by gait perturbations. The maximum amplitude of the CP can be detected over the vertex region. This would be in agreement with an assumption that the CP represent the cerebral processing of impulses originating predominantly from muscle afferents in the leg (Dietz et al., 1985; 1986).

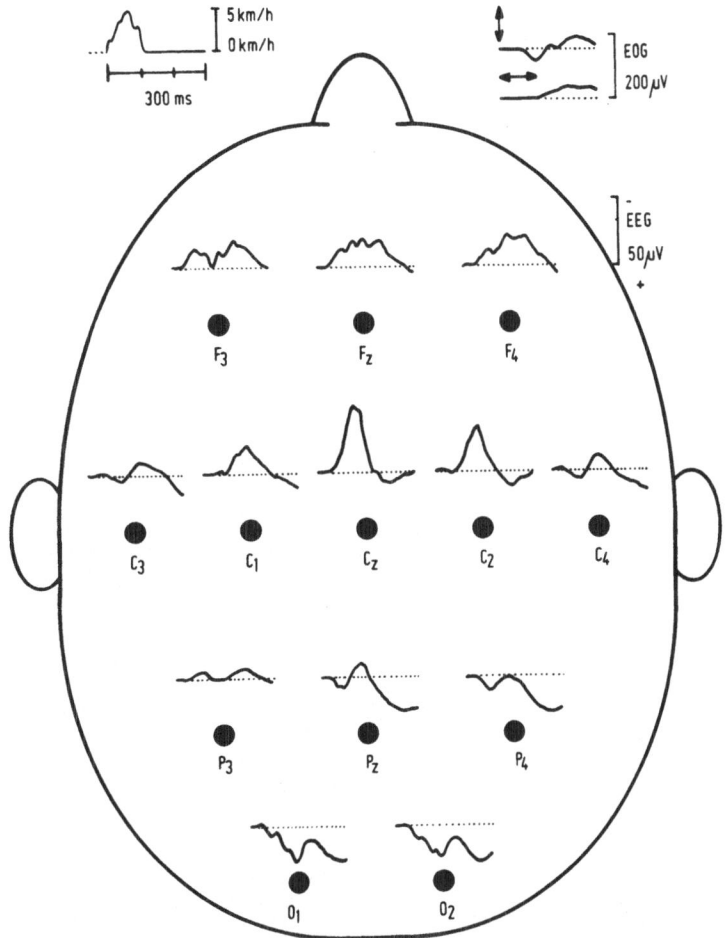

Fig. 4. C.p. (average of 30 trials) evoked by randomly applied treadmill acceleration impulses during stance, recorded at different points over the scalp. Additionally, the electrooculogram is shown.

CONCLUSIONS

Analysis of the EMG responses in the leg following perturbations of posture and gait reveals that monosynaptic stretch reflexes are inhibited during gait and are of minor significance during posture. The functionally essential and appropriate EMG responses are suggested to be mediated predominantly by group II and/or group III leg muscle afferents over a polysynaptic spinal pathway.

The analysis of the cerebral potentials (CP) evoked by tibial nerve stimulation or perturbation during posture and gait provided evidence that transmission to supraspinal motor centers from group I afferents was suppressed. The CP evoked by the perturbation were 3 to 4 times larger compared to those evoked by electrical stimulation. This observation was assumed to be due to cerebral processing of information from leg muscle afferents representing early preparation for a possible fall.

Acknowledgements

We thank Mr S. Fellows for correcting the text. This work was supported by the Deutsche Forschungsgemeinschaft (SFB70 and Be 936/1-2).

REFERENCES

Baldissera, F., Hultborn, H., and Illert, M., 1981, Integration in spinal neuronal systems, in: "Handbook of Physiology. The Nervous System II. Motor Control, Part 1", J. M. Brookhart and V. B. Mountcastle, eds., American Physiological Society, Bethesda.

Dietz, V., and Noth, J., 1978, Spinal stretch reflexes of triceps surae in active and passive movements, J.Physiol., 284:180.

Dietz, V., Noth, J., and Schmidtbleicher, D., 1980, Interaction between pre-activity and stretch reflex in human triceps brachii during landing from forward falls, J.Physiol., 311:113.

Dietz, V., Quintern, J., and Berger, W., 1984, Corrective reactions to stumbling in man: functional significance of spinal and transcortical reflexes, Neurosci.Lett., 44:131.

Dietz, V., Quintern, J., Berger, W., and Schenck, E., 1985, Cerebral potentials and leg muscle EMG responses associated with stance perturbation, Exp.Brain Res., 57:348.

Dietz, V., Quintern, J., and Berger, W., 1985, Afferent control of human stance and gait: evidence for blocking of group I afferents during gait, Exp.Brain Res. (in press).

Dietz, V., Schmidtbleicher, D., and Noth, J., 1979, Neuronal mechanisms of human locomotion, J.Neurophysiol., 42:936.

Morin, C., Katz, R., Mazieres, L., and Pierrot-Desseiligny, E., 1982, Comparison of soleus H-reflex facilitation at the onset of soleus contractions produced voluntarily and during the stance phase of human gait, Neurosci.Lett., 33:47.

Quintern, J., Berger, W., and Dietz, V., 1985, Compensatory reactions to gait perturbations: short and long term effects of neuronal adaptation, Neurosci.Lett. (in press).

Schmidt, R. F., 1971, Presynaptic inhibition in the vertebrate nervous system, Erg.Physiol.Biol.Exp.Pharmakol., 63:20.

Wiesendanger, M., and Miles, T. S., 1982, Ascending pathway of low-threshold muscle afferents to the cerebral cortex and its possible role in motor control, Physiol.Rev., 62:1234.

FACILITATION OF VESTIBULO-MOTOR RESPONSE

BY VOLUNTARY MOVEMENTS IN MAN

B. N. Smetanin, V. Ju. Shlikov, and M. P. Kudinova

Institute for Problems of Information Transmission
USSR Academy of Science
Moscow, USSR

Numerous physiological findings and clinical observations have suggested close association between the vestibular system and the motor
control system. During natural movements this association is organized in
such a way that the vestibular receptors are stimulated due to movements
and the movements, in turn, are influenced by the vestibular input.

Interrelation between the two systems was a subject of a number of
experimental studies performed both with animals and with human subjects.
In addition to many important findings, some contradictory data have been
obtained. For example, Gernand and Gilman (1960) showed that during phasic
electrical stimulation of the motor cortex and the vestibulo-spinal pathways vestibular effects predominated over motor responses. Concerning
tonic vestibular influences, Beritov (1937) argued that the role of neck
and labyrinth receptors is only to assist the activity of coordinatory
structures by increasing their excitability whereas involvement of coordinatory structures into activity is determined by external stimuli.
This conclusion was essentially confirmed by Koella et al. (1956), and
Gernand et al. (1957) who showed that vestibular stimuli resulted in the
changes in muscle tension only when supported by proprioceptive afferentation originating from the extended muscle.

The studies of the effects of various vestibular stimuli on the tendon
jerk and the H-reflex of the leg muscles revealed the increase in the
reflex amplitude in most cases (e.g., Kots and Martjanov, 1967; Hugon et
al., 1971). However, Delwaide and Delbecq (1973) who used both caloric and
electric stimulation of the labyrinth observed the facilitation of the
T-reflex while the H-reflex did not undergo any significant modifications.
Furthermore, vestibular effect on monosynaptic reflex appeared to be
blocked during a local voluntary movement (Kots and Martjanov, 1968).

The above contradictions stimulated this study aimed at elucidating
the mode of interaction between the effects of vestibular stimulation and
some kinds of voluntary movements in the man.

The subjects maintained relaxed standing posture with their eyes
closed, the feet spaced 10-12 cm one from another and placed on the stabilographic platform. The vestibular apparatus was stimulated by a square
pulse of DC of the amplitude of 0.05 to 3.0 mA, the duration of the pulse
being 4 s. The anode was placed over the right mastoid, the cathode over

the medial surface of the right forearm. Vestibulo-motor responses evoked
by electrical stimulation were investigated during quiet standing as well
as during various volitional movements performed after an acoustic
stimulus. These movements included bending down, rising on the tiptoes,
stepping, the Jendrassik manoeuver, etc. 24 adults aged from 25 to 40 were
the subjects in this study.

During quiet stance, the vestibular stimulation resulted in the body
inclination to the right. Minimal currents efficiently inducing these
responses varied among the subjects. For most subjects, they ranged from
0.4 to 0.8 mA but were as large as 1 to 3 mA in some cases.

Figure 1 shows the stabilographic recordings that demonstrate the
changes of supporting forces in the lateral plane during the stimulation
of the right labyrinth. They indicate that in a standing subject the
vestibulo-motor response was directly dependent on the value of the
stimulating current. The current of 0.4 mA induced stimulus-related
stabilographic responses in a few trials only (Figure 1A). The stimulus
intensity of 0.5 mA (Figure 1B) resulted in consistent postural responses
observed all over the trials and the increase of stimulus strength up to
0.9 mA (Figure 1C) was followed by considerable equilibrium disturbances.

Vestibulo-motor responses tested during some voluntary movements
differed considerably from those observed during relaxed standing. Among
various movements tested, the voluntary rising on tiptoes was found to be
most efficient in modifying the vestibulo-motor response. The subjects
were asked to rise rapidly on tiptoes after an acoustic stimulus and then
to return immediately to the initial position. They were trained to perform this movement without large lateral body sways. It was observed that
rising on tiptoes performed during vestibular stimulation resulted in an
increased postural sway, the induced motor response being modified in its
time course compared to that recorded during quiet stance (cf. Figures 1B
and 1E). This difference was most obvious when weak stimuli and rapid
movements were used. In this condition, the body deviation could be
observed with a less intensive labyrinth stimulation (0.1-0.5 mA). The
decrease of the vestibulo-motor threshold was especially pronounced in
those subjects who had relatively high vestibulo-motor thresholds measured
during maintaining a relaxed erect posture.

Furthermore, the vestibulo-motor response was found to depend on the
timing of the voluntary movement relative to the vestibular stimulation.
The largest body deviation occurred when rising on tiptoes was performed
within 100 to 200 ms after the onset of the stimulus (Figure 2). Facilitatory effect of the voluntary movement decreased gradually with the delay

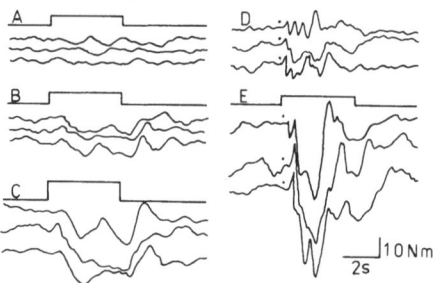

Fig. 1.   Effects of the monoaural vestibular stimulation on the frontal
          stabilogram. (A) 0.4 mA; (B) 0.5 mA; (C) 0.9 mA; (D) rising on
          tiptoes without vestibular stimulation; (E) rising on tiptoes
          during the vestibular stimulation (0.4 mA).

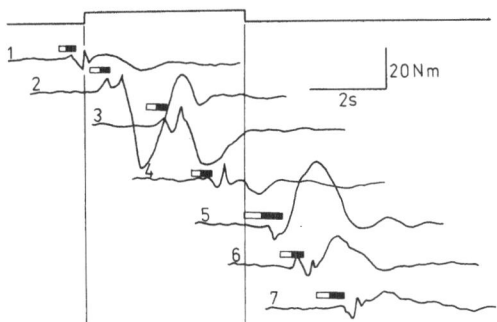

Fig. 2. Lateral stabilographic responses recorded during rising on tiptoes
performed with variable delay after the onset of the galvanic
stimulation. Horizontal bars indicate the timing of the EMG
bursts of the tibialis anterior (open segment) and the soleus
(filled segment) muscles.

between the stimulus and the movement; the increase of the vestibulo-motor
response due to the voluntary movement was small during the last 2 s of the
stimulation. However, when the voluntary movements were initiated simultaneously with the cessation of current the lateral body deviation increased again but the postural sway was directed to the left rather than to
the right.

Further experiments showed that not all the kinds of movements were
equally efficient in the enhancement of the vestibulo-motor response.
Bending down and rising of the forefoot were as efficient as rising on
tiptoes. The forward body inclination, walking, stepping and elevation of
arms were less efficient. Various head movements, the abduction of arms
against elastic resistance as well as isometric contractions of various
muscle groups did not influence the vestibulo-motor response. Involuntary
rising on tiptoes evoked by the bilateral high frequency stimulation
(5 kHz, 0.5 s) of calf muscles did not significantly modify the vestibulo-
motor response.

At the same time, rising on tiptoes as well as other "efficient"
movements performed under the conditions of increased postural stability
(the subject supporting himself against a stable object with the help of
his hands) were followed by a considerable enhancement of the vestibular
response.

Thus the motor response to the electrical stimulation of the labyrinth
that appeared as a lateral body deviation was found to increase when the
subject performed some kinds of voluntary movements. Therefore, the volitional nature of movement is one of the factors determining the observed
enhancement of the vestibulo-motor response. Another possible factor is
related to considerable postural adjustments accompanying the above movements, which necessitate improved postural control. It should be stressed
that any of these factors separately did not determine the described phenomenon.

The data obtained seem to be essential for understanding the function
of the vestibular system in maintaining the equilibrium during various
motor performances. In particular, they suggest that the amount of
vestibular afferentation as well as its contribution to the postural
control could vary depending on the descending neural commands for the
movement initiation. The pattern and the degree of these variations may be
included into the motor program depending on the complexity of the equilibrium maintenance during that particular motor performance.

REFERENCES

Beritov, I. S., 1937, "General Physiology of Muscular and Nervous Systems",
    Biomedgiz, Moscow.
Delwaide, P. J., and Delbecq, P., 1973, Vestibular influences on proprio-
    ceptive reflexes of the lower limb in man, in: "New Developments in
    Electromyography and Clinical Neurophysiology", J. E. Desmedt, ed.,
    vol. 3, Karger, Basel.
Gernand, B. E., and Gilman, S., 1960, Generation of labyrinthine impulses,
    descending vestibular pathways, and modulation of vestibular
    activity by proprioceptive, cerebelar and reticular influences, in:
    "Neural Mechanisms of the Auditory and Vestibular Systems", G. L.
    Rasmussen and W. F. Windle, eds., Springfield, Thomas.
Gernand, B. E., Katsuki, I., and Livingston, R., 1957, Functional organiz-
    ation of descending vestibular influences, J.Neurophysiology,
    20:453.
Hugon, M., Bonnet, M., and Roll, J-P., 1971, Étude des effects moteurs
    d'une stimulation èlectrique vestibulaire chez l'homme, J.Physiol.
    (Paris), 63:15.
Koella, W. P., Nakao, H., Evans, R. L., and Wada, I., 1956, Interaction of
    vestibular and proprioceptive reflexes in decerebrate cat, Amer.J.
    Physiol., 185:607.
Kots, Ya. M., and Martyanov, V. A., 1967, Application of the monosynaptic
    H-reflex to record the effects of electric stimulation of the human
    vestibular apparatus, Cosm.Biol.Med., 3:81 (in Russian).
Kots, Ya. M., and Martyanov, V. A., 1968, Cutting out the vestibulospinal
    influences in the periodic organization of voluntary movement,
    Biofizika, 13:818.

EVALUATION OF MECHANISMS OF POSTURAL REGULATION

BY MEANS OF TIME SERIES ANALYSIS

D. Bräuer and H. Seidel

Central Institute of Occupational Medicine of the GDR
Berlin
East Germany

INTRODUCTION

The displacements of the center of foot pressure which are also called stabilograms, are a reliable measure of postural sway. In accordance with theoretical considerations by Gurfinkel (1973) and experimental studies by Nashner (1971), biomechanical and functional components are assumed to be reflected in the stabilograms. Our experiments aimed at elucidating mechanisms of postural regulation under normal or unusual sensory cues and with different internal levels of conscious control. Earlier investigations (Bräuer and Seidel, 1981) have revealed that stabilograms can well be characterized by autoregressive time series models. In order to analyze postural sway, the decomposition of stabilograms into different components and their parametric characterization appear to be a very promising approach. Another task of our studies was to examine if the decomposition of autoregressive models of higher order into models of the second and the first order can be applied.

METHOD

The data were obtained from two experimental series. In the first series, four male subjects standing with their feet close together were examined in a balanced period design with two repetitions under the following conditions: eyes opened, normal visual field (EO); eyes closed (EC); visual stabilization (VS), i.e., eyes opened and constant visual field; unstable posture (UP), i.e., eyes closed and feet placed on a board with an underlying foam-rubber mat. During all conditions, a light-weight box (30 x 35 x 50 cm) was fixed to the subject's head via a helmet. The box was lined with a chess-board pattern (5 x 5 cm) that was illuminated during VS. A box of identical weight which did not, however, restrict the visual field, was used with EO. In the second series, four highly motivated male subjects from the laboratory staff were instructed to stand with eyes closed, performing two kinds of conscious control of postural sway: utmost attention was focussed on quiet standing (AS) or utmost attention was focussed on quick, speechless counting backward (QC). According to a 4 x 4 Latin square with repetitions, AS and QC were combined with two foot positions - feet together or at an angle of 45 degrees.

The frontal and sagittal stabilograms lasting for 120 seconds were obtained by means of a force platform with a resonant frequency of about 80 Hz, digitized with a sampling rate of 5 per second, and high-pass filtered with a lower cut-off frequency of 0.0875 Hz. The precision of regulation was characterized by means of the standard deviation of the unfiltered and filtered stabilograms. The autoregressive time series modelling of stabilograms (Bräuer and Seidel, 1978) is based on the covariance structure estimated. Models were fitted on the basis of auto-correlation functions, selecting the model with the best goodness of fit (model order limited to 20) by means of the Final Prediction Error Criterion by Akaike (1969). In addition, models of a fixed order were compared. The variance shares accounted for by the model set were estimated for each fitting. The models were decomposed by applying the Bairstow's method to their characteristic polynomials (Sato et al., 1977), including the calculation of the share of variance for all partial models, and the resonant frequency, the phase angle, and the damping factor for the models of second order.

RESULTS

Selected time series parameters of stabilograms obtained in the first experimental series are presented in Table 1. The precision of regulation was different for the experimental conditions. Surprisingly enough, none of the selected parameters indicated significant differences between EC and VS. The variances explained, reflecting the shares to which extent a linear stochastic process is coresponsible for the formation of stabilograms, were highest for EC and VS.

The decomposition of autoregressive models is demonstrated by two sagittal stabilograms obtained in the second series (Figure 1). As becomes obvious from Figure 1, in addition to the two biomechanical main components assumed (Gurfinkel, 1973), further components appeared. However, the components at frequencies of about 0.35 Hz and 1.1 Hz occurred much more frequently than the other ones. The decomposition of each model (7th

Table 1. Mean Values of Selected Time-Series Parameters of Stabilograms

	Experimental conditions				Significant differences				
	1	2	3	4	1/2	1/3	1/4	2/4	3/4
fSDNF	3.58	5.91	6.24	11.01	*	*	*	*	*
fSDFI	2.19	4.45	4.75	9.04	*	*	*	*	*
fVE	.67	.73	.76	.67		*			
fA1	1.14	1.24	1.25	1.02			*	*	*
sSDNF	4.38	5.86	5.54	10.42			*	*	*
sSDFI	1.81	3.31	3.41	8.10	*	*	*	*	*
sVE	.66	.71	.72	.65	*				
sA1	1.03	1.16	1.17	.96	*			*	*

1 = eyes open; 2 = eyes closed; 3 = visual stabilization; 4 = unstable posture; f = frontal; s = sagittal; SDNF = standard deviation of non-filtered stabilograms; SDFI = standard deviation of filtered stabilograms; VE = variance explained by autoregressive models of the 7th order; A1 = first autoregressive coefficient of the autoregressive models of the 7th order.

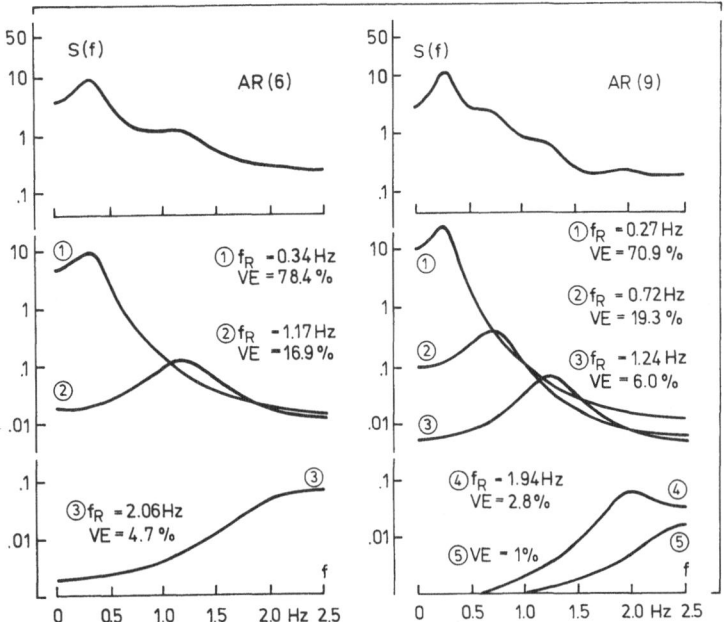

Fig. 1. Decomposition of autoregressive models AR(m) of two sagittal
stabilograms (m = order of the model) in the frequency domain.
The spectra of the autoregressive models (top) are decomposed into
three (bottom, left) and 5 (bottom, right) partial models. All
spectra are normalized. f = resonant frequency; VE = explained
variance.

order) of frontal stabilograms from the first series revealed three partial
models of the 2nd order and one of the 1st order. In the spectrum, they
represent three single peaks within the frequency range and one at the
borderline, respectively. The 1st component was located with its peak at
0.27 Hz, on the average, containing 87.5 ± 7.1% of the total power. The
corresponding data of the 2nd component were 0.97 ± 0.19 Hz and 10 ± 6.8%,
whereas the 3rd component was located at 1.72 ± 0.19 Hz with an amount of
2.2% of the total power. Nearly one third of the partial models of first
order represented a significant share of variance near 0 Hz; the remaining
first order models stood for insignificant high-frequency shares of
variance. The resonant frequencies of the first two components showed
differences between subjects, but no significant differences between the
experimental conditions. However, the remarkably high relative power of
the 1st component with UP went along with a small 2nd component under this
condition. The variance and damping of the first component of frontal
stabilograms were lower, whereas the variance of the second component was
higher with AS than with QC (decomposition of models of the 5th order). In
the sagittal stabilograms, AS was linked with an increased variance of the
2nd component. The level of conscious control did not affect the resonant
frequencies of both components, amounting to 0.38 and 1.3 Hz (frontal) and
0.4 and 1.4 Hz (sagittal).

DISCUSSION

The kind of autoregressive structure of stabilograms during EO may
indicate that a more non-linear control is responsible for the high
precision of regulation with normal sensory cues. VS can happen under real
conditions, e.g., work at height. It went along with a decreased precision

of regulation and changed autoregressive structure. However, on the
average, the sensory conflict between visual, vestibular, and proprioceptive cues did not induce differences, compared to the regulation with
EC, as might be predicted from the results of Vidal et al. (1982).
Obviously, the postural consequences of these conflicting cues depend on
individual factors and the degree of sensory mismatch.

Stabilograms can be regarded as the result of partial processes originating from several generators (Gurfinkel, 1973). The partial models of
the second order might indicate such subsystems. The great constancy of
the partial model with the resonant frequency at about 0.35 Hz suggests an
underlying passive mechanical system possibly identical with one constituent of the displacements of the center of gravity. The part eliminated
by high-pass filtering has to be regarded as another essential constituent.
The rarely appearing partial models are believed to be an expression either
of generators of fluctuant activity or of differences due to the fitting
procedure. The constant resonant frequencies of the two main components
with extremely different levels of conscious control speak in favor of a
biomechanical origin. The "high-frequency" component probably reflects the
activity of leg muscles, increasing with AS. As is suggested by different
results in the frontal and sagittal planes, the interaction of the
different components depends on the direction of sway, too. The present
investigation could not reveal clear differences between the partial models
and their relative spectra in dependence on sensory cues, except from UP.
Thus, the mechanical characteristics of the underlying subsystems themselves, but not of their interrelations, seem to remain constant with EO,
EC, and VS.

REFERENCES

Akaike, H., 1969, Fitting autoregressive models for prediction, Ann.Inst.
    Statist.Math., 21:243.
Bräuer, D., and Seidel, H., 1978, The autoregressive time series modelling
    of stabilograms, Acta Biol.Med.Germ., 37:1221.
Bräuer, D., and Seidel, H., 1981, On the autoregressive structure of
    postural sway, in: "Biomechanics VII-A", A. Morecki, F. Kazimierz,
    K. Krzysztof, and W. Andrzej, eds., Polish Scientific Publishers PWN
    and University Park Press, Warsaw and Baltimore.
Gurfinkel, E. V., 1973, Physical foundations of stabilography,
    Agressologie, 14:9.
Nashner, L. M., 1971, A model describing vestibular detection of body sway
    motion, Acta Oto-Laryngol., 72:429.
Sato, K., Ono, K., Chiba, G., and Fukata, K., 1977, Component activities in
    the autoregressive activity of physiological systems,
    Int.J.Neurosci., 7:239.
Vidal, P. P., Berthoz, A., and Millanvoye, M., 1982, Difference between eye
    closure and visual stabilization in control of posture in man,
    Aviation, Space and Environm.Med., 53:166.

THE EFFECT OF SUPPORT UNLOADING ON CHARACTERISTICS

OF MOTOR CONTROL SYSTEMS ACTIVITY

I. B. Kozlovskaya, I. F. Aslanova, and A. V. Kirenskaya

Institute of Biomedical Problems
Moscow
USSR

Deterioration of the voluntary movement control is a consistent consequence of space flights as well as hypokinesia experiments. Deep changes in a locomotor act structure, disturbances of upright posture, an increased time of motor task performance are always observed even after comparatively short-term exposures to real or simulated hypogravity (Tchkhaidze, 1968; Kubis et al., 1977; Kozlovskaya et al., 1982). The data obtained allowed the suggestion that the support unloading acts as a trigger initiating alteration in the activity of motor control systems under these conditions. As it is known support stimuli play an important role in organization of muscle tonic reactions of posture synergies; the support afferentation is deeply involved in the control of activity of spinal extensor motor neurones. In the absence of support load the tone of gravitational muscles decreases (Mitarai et al., 1978; Kozlovskaya et al., 1983). According to the clinical observations this decrease is in turn the factor that initiates changes in different components of the motor system: muscle afferents and motoneuron entities, reflex mechanisms and trophic apparatus whose activity as shown recently is also determined by the motoneuronal activity (McComas, 1977).

For further understanding of the nature of coordination disturbances, it seemed to be useful to provide a thorough electromyographic study of microgravity effects using the standard test movements as well as standard procedures of quantitative data analysis. The essential part of the work was attributed to the analysis of motor unit activity (MU). Two types of exposure, i.e., to 7-day dry immersion (DI) and to 120-day antiorthostatic bedrest (BR) have been used to simulate effects of short- and long-lasting space flights. It is evident that models under study differ considerably by the degree of support unloading that is quite high in the first case and much less in the second one. Two motor tasks have been used to analyze the microgravity effects on preprogramed and tracking movements control. The test "of precise muscular efforts graduation" (MEG) invented originally by neurologists as a clinical tool assumed to be a good experimental model of preprogramed movements (Burlachkova et al., 1984). Performing this task subjects were asked to execute a series of gradually increasing isometric plantar flexions - from minimal to submaximal one (50-60 kG) with minimal differences in consequent efforts value.

The maintenance of a given level of integrated EMG activity of
m. tibilais anterior (TA) or m. soleus (SOL) and m. gastrocnemius lateralis

(GL) under a situation of visual guidance provided by the arrow of galvano-
meter served as a model of tracking movements. The level of IEMG maintained consisted of about 150 mkV for TA and about 100 mkV for SOL and GL,
being close to the activity level recorded during maintenance of efforts of
7-10% of maximal value. Precise kinematic and electromyographic characteristics of movements have been analyzed before, during and after exposures
to microgravity. The motor unit activity of SOL and GL have been studied
also in the case of tracking performance. The value of effort in this
situation was determined by the recorded on visual display active MU's
number that did not exceed 4-5 for clear identification. As usual, this
value before the exposure was in the range of 5-15% from maximal one.

Simultaneously the function of main proprioceptive inputs - muscle and
support - was assessed with reference to the recruitment function of T- and
H-reflexes of GL or SOL and threshold of the vibrosensitivity of sole
support areas.

The data obtained, demonstrated an obvious decrement in accuracy
control of both movements under study due to both types of weightlessness
simulation, i.e., DI and BR. This decrease in task performance precision
was manifested by a definite increase of values of minimal (absolute threshold) and differential (differential threshold) efforts as well as of
amplitudes of errors and significant decrease of the number of effort
graduations in preprogramed movement task and by a significant rising of
variability of maintained level of IEMG in tracking procedure.

However, the course of alteration of movement characteristics differed
considerably in two conditions under study: in DI the pattern of changes
development was essentially monophasic with peak value on the 3rd day of
exposure. In BR the alterations were developing much more slowly, reveal-
ing clearly two phasic pattern: the first phase lasted till 3-4 weeks of
exposure, the second one occupied the time after 30 days of exposure and
further on.

Both exposures were followed also by a noticeable alteration of parameters of MU activity. The character of changes also revealed great
differences in effects of short- and long-lasting exposures. 7 days DI and
the first phase of BR were characterized by a prominent increase of mean
duration of interspike intervals (ISI), linked to appearance of MU with
unusually low frequency of impulsation, by a significant rising of ISI
variability and also synchronization of MU activity. After 30 days of BR
the mean ISI duration was steadily decreasing, reaching the minimum value
on the 120th day of exposure; the ISI variability at this phase was not
steady, decreasing slightly on the 30-60th day and then rising considerably
again; synchronized activity this time was not evident at all.

The results allow the suggestion that the support unloading,
accompanied by a great reduction of afferent inflow could be considered as
a main "pathogenetic" factor of all changes of movement parameters that
were observed both in short-term as well as in long-term exposures. In
previous studies (Kozlovskaya et al., 1983) we have demonstrated that the
simulated microgravity is followed also by a significant decrease (up to
40% and more) of muscular tone. The course of the coordinatory disorder
development had a close resemblance to that of the muscular tone shift
recorded under the same experimental conditions.

Denervation effects in motor control systems are not studied well
enough. However, it is logically evident that afferent deficiency may
considerably affect the precision of motor performance. Alterations of
muscle properties linked to atonia could become the source of errors in
the first place. The loss of tonic inflow, necessary for maintaining of

certain level motor centers activity could be another factor (Kozlovskaya, 1976). At the same time it is well-known that one of the constant consequences of sensory deficiencies appears to be the hypersensitivity of reflex mechanisms due to an enhancement of excitability of central structures and a decrement of efficiency of inhibitory processes (Kunstman and Orbeli, 1924). The comparative analysis of all data obtained in our experiments allowed the linkage of most of the effects observed in short-term exposures (7 day DI and the first stage of BR) to these shifts in reflex mechanisms excitability. This suggestion is highly supported by data of the MU activity study which revealed at the first stage of microgravity the appearance in ISI hystograms of low frequency MUs that usually are not involved at low levels of muscle efforts, and an increase of ISI

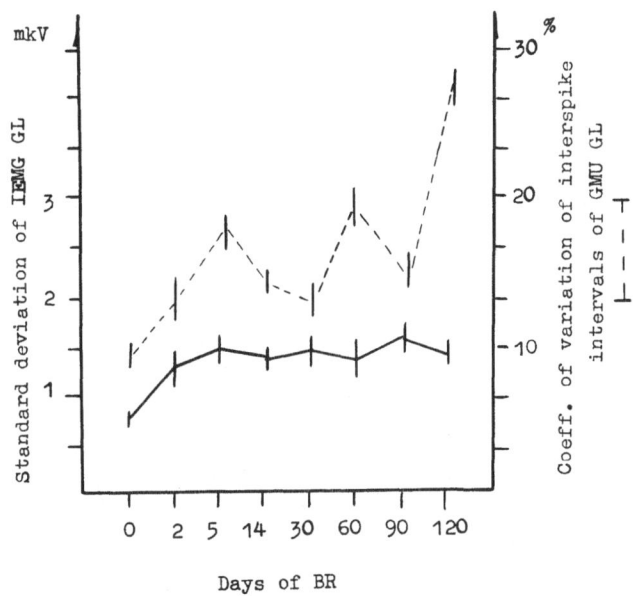

Days of BR

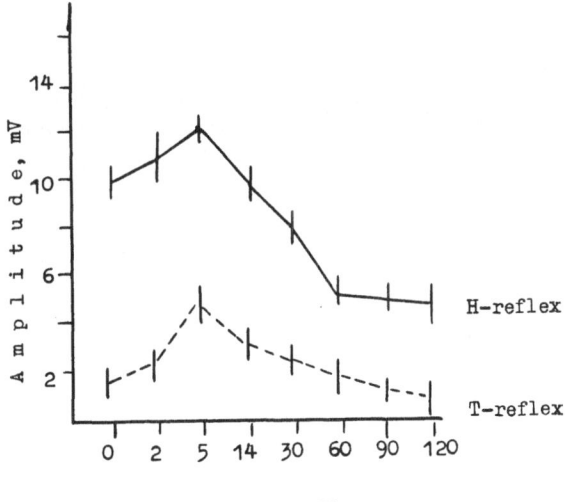

Days of BR

Fig. 1. Characteristics of IEMG, ISI variability (upper part) and T- and H-reflexes amplitudes (lower part) at different time intervals of BR.

variability, which could be most probably a result of inhibitory deficiency going along with excitability increase. It is known that the Renshaw's inhibitory systems play an important role in possessing stability of motoneurons rhythmic activity. The same signs of an increased excitability of motoneuronal populations at the above mentioned stage of microgravity have been revealed by the results of studies of T- and H-reflexes characteristics, demonstrating clearly a decrease of the amplitudes of both reflexes in 7 day DI and even more pronounced during the first 15-30 days of BR (Figure 1). At the second stage of BR the hypersensitivity marks diminished gradually pointing out to the development of other processes, linked probably to some alterations of properties of neuro-muscular peripheria.

REFERENCES

Burlatchkova, N. I., Kozlovskaya, I. B., Gurskaya, N. Z., and Markova, E. D., 1984, Characteristics of tracking and programed movements in various disturbances of cerebello-cortical system, in: "Modern Aspects of Cerebellar Functions", Acad. Sci. Arm. SSR., Erevan (in Russian).

Kozlovskaya, I. B., 1976, Afferent control of voluntary movements, Nauka, Moscow (in Russian).

Kozlovskaya, I. B., Aslanova, I. F., Grigorieva, L. S., and Kreidich, Yu. V., 1982, Experimental analysis of motor effects of weightlessness, A Suppl.Physiologist, 25:S49.

Kozlovskaya, I. B., Aslanova, I. F., Barmin, V. A., Grigorieva, L. S., Gevlich, G. I., Kirenskaya, A. V., and Sirota, M. G., 1983, The nature and characteristics of gravitational ataxia, A Suppl. Physiologist, 26:S108.

Kubis, J. F., McLaughlin, E. J., Jackson, J. M., Rusnak, R., McBride, G., and Saxon, S. V., 1977, Task and work performance on skylab missions 2, 3 and 4: time and motion study experiment M-151, in: "Biomedical Results from Skylab", R. S. Johnson and L. F. Dietlein, eds., NASA SP-377.

Kunstman, K. I., and Orbelli, L. A., 1924, About consequences of deafferentation of the hind limbs in dogs, Izv.Petrogr.Inst.im A.F. Lesgafta, 9:187.

McComas, A. J., 1977, "Neuromuscular Function and Disorders", Butterworths, London-Boston.

Mitarai, G., Mano, T., Mori, M., and Jamasaki, J., 1978, Compensatory leg muscle function shift during adaptation to simulated weightlessness, XXYI Intern.Congr.Aerosp.Med., London Sept. 4-8.

Tchkhaidze, L. V., 1968, Coordination of voluntary movements in man in space flight conditions, Nauka, Moscow.

SECTION V
LOCOMOTION

ACTIVITY OF VENTRAL SPINOCEREBELLAR TRACT NEURONS CHRONICALLY

RECORDED IN THE SPINAL CORD OF AWAKE, FREELY MOVING CATS

C. L. Cleland and J. A. Hoffer

Department of Clinical Neurosciences
Faculty of Medicine, University of Calgary
Calgary, Alberta, Canada

INTRODUCTION

The cerebellum receives information about the hindlimb from mossy and climbing fiber pathways. One of the mossy fiber pathways, the ventral spinocerebellar tract (VSCT), arises from large neurons in the intermediate and ventral portions of the spinal cord. VSCT axons cross the midline, ascend in the ventrolateral funiculus, and terminate bilaterally in the cerebellum (Oscarsson, 1965).

Electrophysiological investigations of VSCT neurons in anesthetized or reduced cat preparations have demonstrated convergence of sensory, descending and interneuronal input (see Bloedel and Courville, 1981). VSCT neurons can receive monosynaptic and polysynaptic excitation from Ia and Ib afferents arising from several muscles. Most VSCT neurons are also excited by contralateral flexor reflex afferents (FRAs) and inhibited by ipsilateral FRAs. Descending excitation is provided by the motor cortex, the red nucleus, Deiter's nucleus and the reticular formation. Polysynaptic inhibition can also be evoked by the same pathways that provide excitation. This extensive knowledge obtained from experiments in anesthetized and reduced preparations, however, is insufficient to predict the normal strength and pattern of different inputs in the conscious, behaving animal.

During locomotion or scratching in decerebrated cats, modulation of the activity of VSCT neurons persisted after deafferentation (Arshavsky et al., 1972), elimination of modulation in descending pathways by cerebellectomy (Arshavsky et al., 1972), and cooling the spinal cord caudal to L5 (Arshavsky et al., 1984). Therefore, spinal mechanisms rostral to L5 are sufficient to rhythmically modulate VSCT activity. However, these results did not elucidate the role of descending and sensory convergence in the normal cat.

Three general alternative hypotheses on the function of the VSCT have been proposed. Individual VSCT neurons may encode information regarding 1) sensory receptor activity (Oscarsson, 1965), 2) transmission in interneuronal pathways (Lundberg, 1971; Lindstrom, 1973; Arshavsky et al., 1984) or 3) "efference copy" of motoneurons (Lundberg, 1971). Current knowledge about the VSCT is not sufficient to distinguish among these hypotheses. The known connections of VSCT neurons are consistent with all three hypotheses and although Arshavsky and colleagues showed that interneuronal activity alone was sufficient to modulate the activity of VSCT neurons, they did not address the contributions from descending and sensory pathways. Consequently, we have developed a method for recording the natural activity of VSCT neurons in freely moving cats in order to test these three hypotheses.

METHODS

Four cats were trained to walk on a motorized treadmill, stand quietly on four pedestals and tolerate passive manipulations of the limbs. The paw shake, scratching, flexion withdrawal reflexes and various voluntary limb movements were evoked without training.

A variety of recording and stimulating devices were chronically implanted in the spinal cord and left hindlimb. The design, location and recording procedures are described in detail elsewhere (Cleland and Hoffer, 1986; Hoffer and Loeb, 1980). Briefly, six to twelve floating microelectrodes, similar to the "hatpin" microelectrodes used previously to record from single units in the ventral roots (Hoffer et al., 1981) or dorsal root ganglia (Loeb et al., 1985), were implanted in the lateral funiculi of spinal cord segments T13-L2. Recording/stimulating surface electrodes were implanted intra- or extradurally on opposite sides of the thoracic spinal cord. Muscle electromyograms (EMGs) were recorded from six hindlimb muscles with bipolar electrodes. Joint angles were measured by implanting length transducers across the ankle, knee and hip joints. Muscle nerves were stimulated through cuff electrodes implanted on the femoral, sciatic and hamstring nerves. Fluids and drugs were administered through a catheter in the external jugular vein. The leads from each device were routed subcutaneously to an external connector and signals were transmitted through a 40-conductor ribbon cable.

After the cat recovered from surgery, the microelectrodes were scanned daily to determine if any discriminable units were present. If a microelectrode recorded the activity of a unit that could be tentatively identified as a VSCT neuron, data were collected from the implanted transducers while the cat performed his repertoire of motor tasks. Afterwards, the cat was anesthetized and the receptive fields of the recorded VSCT neuron were examined.

RESULTS

Ninety discriminable units were recorded from 97 microelectrodes. The shape and amplitude of individual unitary action potentials ranged from 20-150 μV and remained stable even during vigorous movements. Individual units could often be followed for 2-12 consecutive days.

The VSCT is the only crossed ascending hindlimb pathway that receives extensive monosynaptic excitation from hindlimb group I muscle afferents (see Cleland and Hoffer, 1986). Therefore, units were identified as VSCT neurons if they were excited at short latency by low-intensity electrical stimulation of hindlimb nerves and had an ascending projection.

Seven of the recorded single units were identified as VSCT neurons. The average intensity of electrical stimulation required to excite these neurons was 1.25×T (Twitch threshold; range 0.8- 2.3×T). Variability in the latency excluded primary sensory afferents. An ascending projection extending as far as the mid-thoracic spinal cord was demonstrated for 3/7 neurons. Two of these were antidromically excited by electrical stimulation through the thoracic spinal cord surface electrodes. Spike-triggered averaging of the neurogram recorded by the surface electrodes was used to demonstrate the ascending projection of the third neuron. The conduction velocities of these three neurons were 41, 81 and 139 m/s. It is likely that the other four neurons were also ascending tract neurons since they had distal receptive fields and were recorded in the L2-L3 lateral funiculi.

The synaptic properties of the VCST neurons were consistent with the literature (Bloedel and Courville, 1981). Three of four VSCT neurons tested for group I muscle afferent input from more than one hindlimb nerve demonstrated convergence. The threshold for excitation by electrical stimulation was consistently increased by pentobarbital anesthesia. One of two VSCT neurons tested was excited by electrical stimulation of the contralateral sural nerve. These features support their identification as VSCT neurons.

The activity of all seven VSCT neurons was modulated during normal behavior. Figure 1 is an example showing the activity of a VSCT neuron during a voluntary movement. As the cat gradually shifted from a lying to standing position, extensor muscle EMG and the activity of the VSCT neuron increased in parallel. When the cat briefly lifted his foot off the ground, shown by the interruption in the ground contact bar, the activity of the neuron decreased to zero and only resumed when contact returned. Note that the decrease in activity began closer to footlift than to the flexor EMG responsible for the movement. From this brief segment, it appears that the activity of this VSCT neuron was correlated with a stance-related variable, such as contact force. However, because contact force covaries with other variables, it is impossible to decide from these data alone which variables were best correlated with VSCT activity.

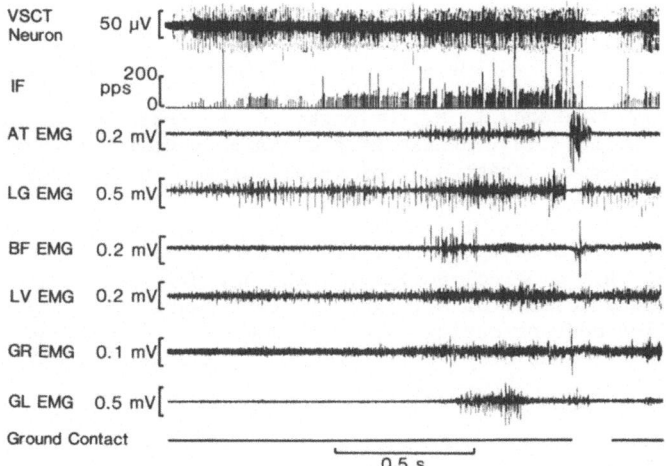

Fig. 1. Natural activity of a VSCT neuron during a voluntary movement. The top trace shows the raw activity recorded by the floating microelectrode. The second trace is the instantaneous frequency of the neuron with the larger of the two action potentials visible in the raw record. The few exceptionally high rates were probably false acceptances of spikes generated by the smaller neuron. The next six traces are the EMGs from the anterior tibial (AT), lateral gastrocnemius (LG), biceps femoris (BF), lateral vastus (LV), gracilis (GR) and gluteus medius (GL) muscles. The bottom trace indicates the period of time that the left hind paw maintained contact with the ground, which was determined from video tape records.

There were differences in the patterns of activity of the VSCT neurons. Six were most strongly modulated during changes in muscle length or force. Five of these were active during the extension phase and the other was active during the flexion phase of locomotion. The seventh VSCT neuron was excited only by light cutaneous stimulation. In future experiments, we will investigate whether these differences reflect distinct functional classes of VSCT neurons.

CONCLUSIONS

We have successfully recorded the activity of VSCT neurons in the spinal cord of awake cats during unrestrained movements. Previous studies of VSCT neurons were performed in anesthetized or decerebrated cats because of the difficulties in recording from the spinal cord of awake, behaving animals (see Cleland and Hoffer, 1986). The use of floating microelectrodes has allowed us to overcome the recording difficulties and obtain stable records from spinal neurons. Although our data are still too preliminary to determine whether the activity of VSCT neurons is better correlated with sensory, motor or interneuronal activity, in future experiments we hope to determine the nature of the information normally conveyed by the VSCT to the cerebellum.

Acknowledgments

We thank E. Ebly and T. Leonard for assistance. Funds were provided by the Alberta Heritage Foundation for Medical Research and the Medical Research Council of Canada.

REFERENCES

Arshavsky, Y. I., Berkinblit, M. B., Gelfand, I. M., Orlovsky, G. N., and Fukson, O. I., 1972, Activity of the neurones of the ventral spinocerebellar tract during locomotion of cats with deafferentated hind limbs, Biofizika (engl.trans.), 17:1169.
Arshavsky, Y. I., Gelfand, I. M., Orlovsky, G. N., Pavlova, G. A., and Popova, L. B., 1984, Origin of signals conveyed by the ventral spino-cerebellar tract and spino-reticulo-cerebellar pathway, Exp.Brain Res., 54:426.
Bloedel, J. R. and Courville, J., 1981, Cerebellar afferent systems, in: "Handbook of Physiology, Vol. II, Motor Control," V. B. Brooks, ed., American Physiological Society, Bethesda, Maryland.
Cleland, C. L. and Hoffer, J. A., 1986, Activity patterns of spinocerebellar neurons during normal locomotion. Proceedings of the symposium "Neurobiology of Vertebrate Locomotion," Stockholm, Sweden, Macmillan Press (in press).
Hoffer, J. A. and Loeb, G. E., 1980, Implantable electrical and mechanical interfaces with nerve and muscle, Annals Biomed.Engr., 8:351.
Hoffer, J. A., O'Donovan, M. J., Pratt, C. A., and Loeb, G. E., 1981, Discharge patterns of hindlimb motoneurons during normal cat locomotion, Science, 213:466.
Lindstrom, S., 1973, Recurrent inhibition from motor axon collaterals of Ia inhibitory pathways in the spinal cord of the cat, Acta Physiol. Scand.Suppl., 392:1.
Loeb, G. E., Hoffer, J. A., and Pratt, C. A., 1985, Activity of spindle afferents from cat anterior thigh muscles. I. Identification and patterns during normal locomotion, J.Neurophysiol., 54:549.
Lundberg, A., 1971, Function of the ventral spinocerebellar tract. A new hypothesis, Exp.Brain Res., 12:317.
Oscarsson, O., 1965, Functional organization of the spinocerebellar and cuneocerebellar tracts, Physiol.Rev., 45:495.

ACTIVITY PATTERNS OF IDENTIFIED ALPHA MOTONEURONS TO CAT ANTERIOR

THIGH MUSCLES DURING NORMAL WALKING AND FLEXOR REFLEXES

G. E. Loeb*, J. A. Hoffer, N. Sugano, W. B. Marks
M. J. O'Donovan, and C. A. Pratt

Laboratory of Neural Control
National Institutes of Health
Bethesda, MD

INTRODUCTION

The organization of the motor apparatus into anatomically and functionally defined pools of regularly recruited motor units derives from
some of the earliest and most enduring observations of neurophysiology.
In recent years, there has been much productive research concentrated on
discovering the anatomical bases of this organization in the spinal cord
circuitry and the properties of the final common pathway, the alpha motoneurons themselves (for review, see Burke, 1981a). However, almost all of
the direct evidence for the function of this system has been derived from
experiments on reduced or anesthetized animals and on human subjects performing highly constrained and artificial motor tasks.

Over the past few years, we have been able to obtain recordings in
intact, normally walking cats from single ventral root axons projecting to
identified hindlimb muscles. This paper presents a brief summary of the
most salient features noted in these studies (full reports are in preparation; abstracts of these data have been presented elsewhere). In general,
the results have confirmed the broad outlines of current motor recruitment
theories, while emphasizing new or overlooked features such as the importance of rate modulation and the complexities of multifunctional muscles.

METHODS

Seventeen adult cats were implanted chronically with a variety of
recording electrodes and transducers, using general anesthesia and aseptic
surgical techniques. Data from a total of 164 axons in the fifth lumbar
ventral roots (L5 VR) were recorded during normal motor behavior at 1-10
weeks postoperatively, using a 40 pin percutaneous connector and multichannel analog and video recording equipment to provide correlary kinesio-
logical information from the hindlimb.

*Correspondence: G. E. Loeb, National Institutes of Health, Bldg. 36,
 Rm. 5A29, 9000 Rockville Pike, Bethesda, MD 20892

Unit Recording and Identification

Up to twelve floating microelectrodes were implanted in L5 VR via
a small laminotomy. Each electrode consisted of a 50 micron shaft of
80-20% Pt-Ir alloy welded to a twisted pair of very flexible, 25 micron
diameter, gold wires, in turn welded to stranded stainless steel cable for
percutaneous exit, with the entire assembly overcoated with 15 microns of
Parylene-C polymer (Loeb et al., 1977), and strain-relieved by passing
through a short piece of silicone rubber tubing affixed to the dorsal
spines. Once implanted, each electrode was tested daily for impedance
(typically 80-220 kilohms at 1 kHz) and the presence of discriminable
single unit action potentials during walking on a treadmill.

Spike-triggered signal averaging was used successfully on 43 units to
identify both the efferent conduction velocity and the muscle of destin-
ation. The femoral nerve (to which about half of the L5 segment projects)
was chronically instrumented with a nerve cuff electrode that provided two
adjacent tripolar recording sites for averaging the efferent action potentials from the triggering unit (Hoffer et al., 1981). The complete motor
projections of the femoral nerve distal to the cuff include the monartic-
ular vasti (lateralis-VL, medialis-VM, and intermedius-VI) and biarticular
rectus femoris-RF and sartorius (pars medialis-SA-m and anterior-SA-a), all
of which were chronically implanted with bipolar recording electrodes.
Spike-triggered averaging of all of these EMG records usually revealed one
predominant record, by which we identified the muscle innervated by the
triggering unit.

Neurokinesiological Data Processing

The locomotor cycle was recorded by a high resolution video system
with a time code to permit correlation with the analog signals recorded on
18-track FM tape (DC-10 kHz). All unit identification and analysis was
performed off-line on the same recorded sequences, using conventional
spike-discrimination equipment (Bak and Schmidt, 1977) and analog rectifi-
cation and integration of EMG activity (Bak and Loeb, 1979) prior to digiti-
zation and computer analysis. For each motor unit, covariances were calculated between the instantaneous frequencygram (inverse of interspike
interval) and the complete set of EMG signals (digitally smoothed with
about 30 msec time-constant).

The limb was also implanted with length gauges (saline-filled lengths
of elastic silicone rubber tubing with electrodes in each end; Loeb et al.,
1980) across the vasti muscle group (pure knee extensors) and RF-SA-a group
(knee extensors plus hip flexors). These records plus their electronic
time derivatives (velocity) are shown in the figures, along with the output
of an implanted tendon strain gauge on the patellar ligament (Walmsley et
al., 1978), where all muscles except SA-m insert.

A nerve cuff electrode on the saphenous nerve was electronically
stimulated with single current pulses (0.1 msec duration, 1.1-10 times
threshold for group I fibers) to provide segmental cutaneous perturbations
at random points in the step cycles. The prestimulus controls and flexor
reflex responses of the various muscles and 11 motor axons were ordered
into rasters on the basis of the phase in the step cycle at which each
stimulus occurred (Abraham et al., 1985).

FINDINGS

Figures 1 and 2 show typical sets of tracings of unit frequencygrams
plus rectified EMG from various muscles, including that innervated by the

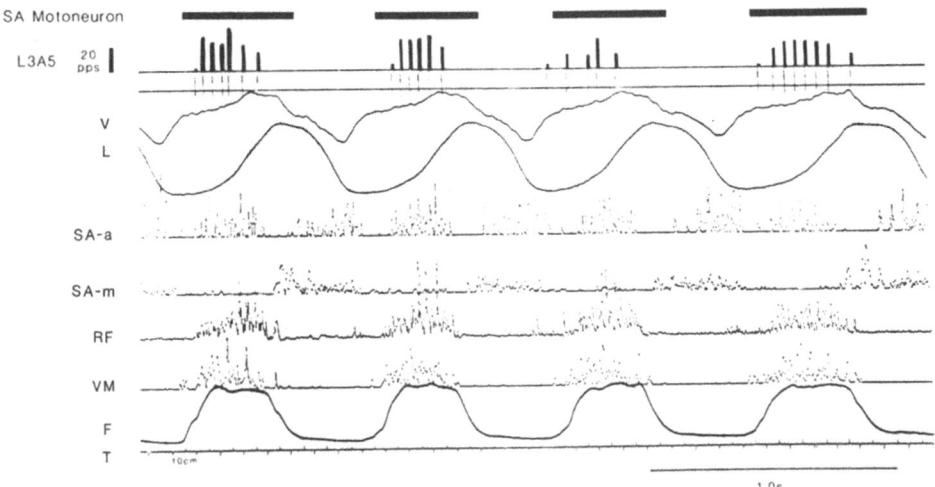

Fig. 1. Activity of a ventral root axon projecting to anterior sartorius muscle, during four normal walking step cycles (heavy bars denote stance phase). Traces from top down: frequency of unit firing, window discriminator output, velocity of muscle (stretch upward), length of muscle, rectified EMG integrated into 2 msec bins from anterior sartorius, medial sartorius, rectus femoris, and vastus medialis muscles, force output at patellar ligament strain gauge, and treadmill speed. Note unit activity only during stance phase EMG activity of parent muscle SA-a.

unit, and length and force records during unperturbed treadmill walking. All of the motor units tended to be recruited in a single burst of activity each step cycle, beginning firing at about 8-15 pps whenever the amplitude of the parent muscle EMG exceeded a threshold that was typical for each unit and relatively independent of walking speed. The unit firing rate was always well-modulated in close correlation with parent muscle EMG, and could approach 50 pps even for first-recruited, presumably slow-twitch motoneurons. Units recruited at less than 50% of the peak EMG level tended to have axon conduction velocities of 50-90 m/s (8 of 10 units) whereas those recruited above 50% had axon conduction velocities of 90-120 m/s (14 of 18 units). Initial doublets (interspike intervals of less than 20 msec at the beginning of recruitment) were seen in only four out of 51 units.

The two motoneurons shown in the figures are of particular interest because they have typical single activity bursts per step cycle despite the fact that their parent muscle, SA-a, had two EMG bursts per step cycle. Unit L3A5 in Figure 1 was active only during and in proportion to the stance phase muscle activity, whereas unit L2A42 in Figure 2 was active only during and in proportion to the swing phase muscle activity. Even when the EMG in the opposite phase exceeded levels usually associated with unit recruitment, all 13 motoneurons projecting to either part of the sartorius muscle maintained their phase-dependent selectivity without exception. For the phase of EMG recruitment associated with the unit discharge, the covariance of unit activity and EMG amplitude was just as high as for units projecting to unifunctional muscles, typically accounting for 88-95% of the variance of unitary spike rates.

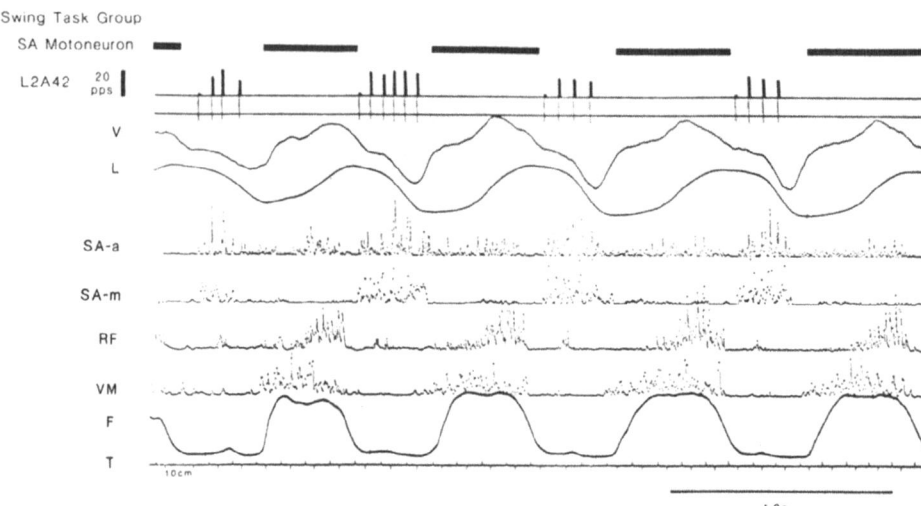

Fig. 2. Activity of a ventral root axon projecting to SA-a muscle during normal walking, traces as in Figure 1. Note unit activity only during swing phase EMG activity of parent muscle SA-a.

During reflex responses elicited by saphenous nerve stimulation, all of the bifunctional muscles (SA-a, SA-m, and RF, which is normally active only during stance for slow walking) and their motor axons were recruited quite homogeneously. Six units studied thoroughly under this paradigm (three from SA-a and three from RF) all responded with typical flexor muscle responses including short latency (5–15 msec) and/or long latency (20–35 msec) excitatory responses that were complexly gaited in both the stance and swing phases of locomotion. In particular, units projecting to bifunctional muscles that were normally active only during the stance (extensor) phase produced reflex responses that were typical of flexor muscles, whereas units projecting to pure extensor muscles (vasti) produced typical extensor reflexes, typified by inhibition and occasional late excitatory rebound.

CONCLUSIONS

These studies have confirmed many important concepts of motor control derived from reduced preparations, while at the same time pointing out important details and exceptions that have not been seen in such preparations:

1. Motor units are recruited in a regular and reproducible manner, with recruitment order at least loosely correlated with the conduction velocity of the motor axons (see Henneman and Mendell, 1981, for review).

2. Activity patterns tend to be much more smoothly and broadly modulated in the normal cat than in decerebrate preparations, where initial doublet activity followed by relatively stereotyped activity at a "preferred firing rate" is the usual pattern (Zajac and Young, 1980).

3. The main difference between early recruited (presumably slow twitch, fatigue resistant) and late recruited (high threshold, presumably fast, fatiguable) motor units is in the proportion of the time that they are active, rather than in the particular spike rates or

patterns generated. This is in contrast to earlier findings regarding 'tonic' vs. 'phasic' patterns reported for low and high-threshold units in reduced preparations (Granit et al., 1957), and it has important implications for theories regarding plasticity of muscle unit properties (see e.g. Salmons and Vrbova, 1969; reviewed by Burke, 1981b).

4. The very close covariance between unit spike rates and EMG amplitude suggests that all members of each functional recruitment group receive the same net input signal, differing only in amplitude and/or threshold of response. Conversely, EMG signals recorded and processed in the manner employed here appear to provide a remarkably good indication of this command signal, including fine details of temporal modulation resulting from the interaction of the locomotor pattern generator and various descending and segmental influences.

5. Bifunctional muscles such as anterior sartorius may be divided functionally into separately recruited groups, perhaps related to kinematically opposite conditions such as active lengthening during stance phase and active shortening during swing (see Loeb, 1985).

6. The above-noted task-dependent recruitment groups can be over-ridden during different motor tasks such as the flexor reflex, where all units with a similar mechanical action (in this case, hip flexion) were recruited together regardless of their locomotor task group participation.

REFERENCES

Abraham, L. D., Marks, W. B., and Loeb, G. E., 1985, The distal hindlimb musculature of the cat: Cutaneous reflexes during locomotion, Exp.Brain Res., 58:594-603.

Bak, M. J., and Loeb, G. E., 1979, A pulsed integrator for EMG analysis, Electroenceph.Clin.Neurophysiol., 47:738-741.

Bak, M. J., and Schmidt, E. M., 1977, An improved time-amplitude window discriminator, IEEE BME, 24:486-489.

Burke, R. E., 1981a, Motor units: Anatomy, physiology and functional organization, in: "Handbook of Physiology, Section I. The Nervous System III. Motor Systems," B. V. Brooks, ed., Am.Physiol.Soc., pp.345-422, Washington, DC.

Burke, R. E., 1981b, The stability of motor unit types in response to altered functional demand: Hypertrophy, atrophy and reinnervation models, in: "Mechanisms of Muscle Adaptation to Functional Requirements," F. Gaba, G. Marechal, O. Takacs, eds., pp.45-56, Akademiai Kiado, Budapest.

Granit, R., Phillips, C. G. Skoglund, S., and Steg, G., 1957, Differentiation of tonic from phasic ventral horn cells by stetch, pinna and crossed extensor reflexes, J.Neurophysiol., 20:470-481.

Henneman, E., and Mendell, L. M., 1981, Functional organization of motoneuron pool and its inputs, in: "Handbook of Physiology, Section II. The Nervous System, Volume II. Motor Control, Part 2," V. B. Brooks, ed., Am.Physiol.Soc., pp.423-507, Bethesda, MD.

Hoffer, J. A., Loeb, G. E., and Pratt, C. A., 1981, Single unit conduction velocities from averaged nerve cuff electrode records in freely moving cats, J.Neurosci.Meth., 4:211-225.

Loeb, G. E., 1985, Motoneuron task groups - coping with kinematic heterogeneity, J.Exp.Biol., 115:137-146.

Loeb, G. E., Bak, M. J., Salcman, M., and Schmidt, E. M., 1977, Parylene as a chronically stable, reproducible microelectrode insulator, IEEE-BME, 24:121-128.

Loeb, G. E., Walmsley, B., and Duysens, J., 1980, Obtaining proprioceptive information from natural limbs: Implantable transducers vs. somatosensory neuron recordings, in: "Physical Sensors for Biomedical

Applications. Proc. of Workshop on Solid State Physical Sensors for Biomedical Application," M. R. Neuman et al., eds., CRC Press, Inc., Boca Raton.

Salmons, S., and Vrbova, G., 1969, The influence of activity on some contractile characteristics of mammalian fast and slow muscles, J.Physiol.(Lond.), 201:535-549.

Walmsley, B., Hodgson, J. A., and Burke, R. E., 1978, Forces produced by medial gastrocnemius and soleus muscles during locomotion in freely moving cats, J.Neurophysiol., 41:1203-1216.

Zajac, F. E., and Young, J. L., 1980, Discharge properties of hindlimb motoneurons in decerebrate cats during locomotion induced by mesencephalic stimulation, J.Neurophysiol., 43:1221-1235.

ANTIDROMIC DISCHARGES OF PRIMARY AFFERENTS DURING LOCOMOTION

R. Dubuc, J. -M. Cabelguen, and S. Rossignol*

Centre de Recherche en Sciences Neurologiques
Département de Physiologie, Faculté de Médecine
Université de Montréal, Montréal, Québec, Canada

It is generally recognized that there are mechanisms in the spinal cord by which the primary afferent terminals may be subjected to depolarizing actions. The latter are believed to serve as a substrate for presynaptic inhibition (Eccles et al., 1963). From a functional standpoint, there are indications that presynaptic inhibition might occur during rhythmic movements. Indeed, during fictive locomotion and scratching in the cat, primary afferent terminals have been shown to be subjected to both tonic and phasic depolarizing actions of central origin (Bayev and Kostyuk, 1982a,b). While reassessing such presynaptic mechanisms during locomotion, we have confirmed the presence of phasic fluctuations of dorsal root potential (Dubuc et al., 1985) and have further recorded a number of units discharging antidromic action potentials in cut dorsal root filaments (Dubuc et al., 1986). In the present paper, we will report primarily on these antidromic discharges as they provide a means of looking at polarizing actions exerted at the single unit level.

Ten cats were decorticated (Perret and Cabelguen, 1980) under methohexital sodium anesthesia and subsequently paralyzed with gallamine triethiodide (10 mg/kg repeated when needed). Motor nerves of the left hindlimb were dissected and recorded with Ag/AgCl electrodes in a pool of warm paraffin oil. An extensive laminectomy (L3 to S2) was performed and the spinal cord was covered with paraffin oil. Special care was taken to maintain the oil temperature at 38°C with a feedback controlled heating element. Fictive locomotion occurred spontaneously or, in a few cases, was initiated by short trains of stimulation applied to one lumbar dorsal root. In some preparations, the spinal cord was transected at the last thoracic level (Th13) and fictive locomotion was induced by an i.v. injection of nialamide (50 mg/kg) and L-DOPA (80 mg/kg). Two of the decorticate cats were not paralyzed and allowed to walk on a treadmill belt. In these animals, the locomotor discharges were recorded with percutaneous electrodes inserted in muscles of both hindlimbs.

Small dorsal root filaments were cut a few milimeters proximal to the ganglion; they were carefully dissected and mounted on Ag/AgCl electrodes (Figure 1). Interestingly, most filaments showed spontaneous antidromic discharges and in such cases, the filaments were further dissected until

---

*Correspondence to: Dr Serge Rossignol, at above address.

single units were recorded. Since antidromic discharges could be recorded
in filaments cut several hours previously, it is unlikely that they represent injury discharges.

A total of 194 units were recorded and 40% of those showed bursts of
activity which were related to the efferent locomotor rhythm. Figure 1
illustrates one such unit, recorded from the proximal stump of a cut dorsal
root filament during fictive locomotion in the decorticate cat. The discharges occur in bursts at fixed times during the locomotor cycle. The
unit starts discharging near the onset of activity in the hip flexor muscle
nerve (iSartL) and ceases firing at the beginning of activity in the hip
extensor muscle nerve (iSmA). Similar antidromic discharges related to the
ongoing rhythm were also recorded in the spinal cat during DOPA-induced
fictive locomotion. It is noteworthy that in both the decorticate and the
spinal cat preparation, unit discharges could occur in different phases of
the locomotor cycle (see also Dubuc et al., 1986).

The discharge pattern of the other units (60%) was not related to the
efferent locomotor activity. Figure 2A illustrates the antidromic discharges recorded from a cut dorsal root filament of L6 in the paralyzed
spinal cat during DOPA-induced locomotion. The unit has a tonic discharge
pattern which is clearly not modulated by the ongoing locomotor rhythm.
Interestingly however, the discharge of this particular unit was markedly
influenced by exteroceptive stimulation as shown in Figure 2B. In this
case, as the contralateral hindlimb was repetitively subjected to passive
flexion and extension at the hip joint, the unit increased its discharge

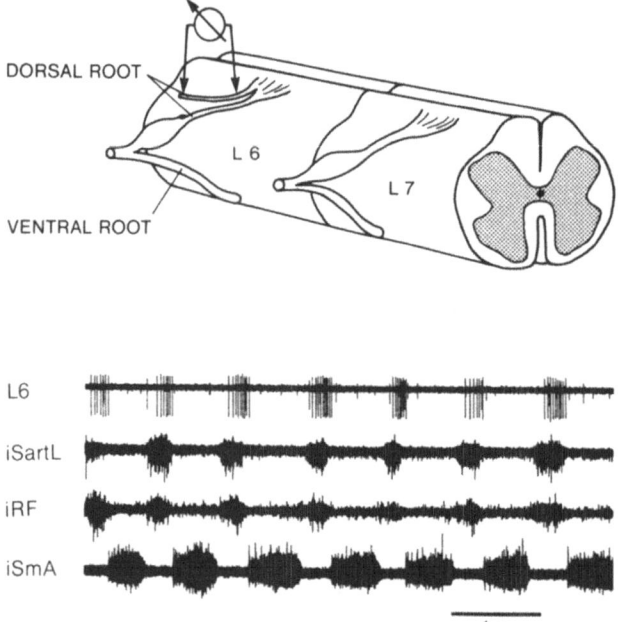

Fig. 1. Top: Schematic representation of the dorsal root filament
         recording procedure. Note that the rest of the spinal roots were
         in continuity with the periphery. Bottom: Antidromic discharges
         recorded from the proximal stump of a cut dorsal root filament at
         the 6th lumbar segment (L6). The fictive locomotor discharges are
         recorded from nerves of the ipsilateral hindlimb: the sartorius
         lateralis (iSartL), the rectus femoris (iRF) and the semimembran-
         osus anterior (iSmA).

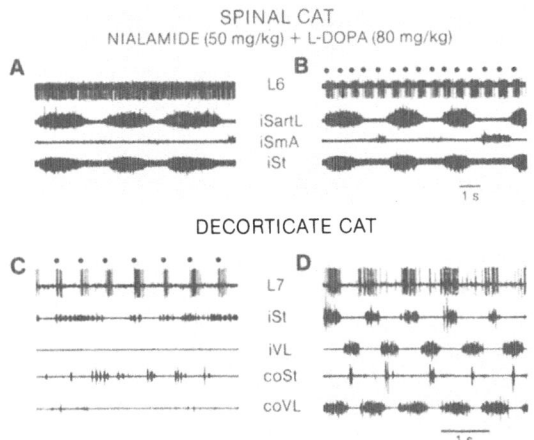

SPINAL CAT
NIALAMIDE (50 mg/kg) + L-DOPA (80 mg/kg)

A   B

L6
iSartL
iSmA
iSt

1 s

DECORTICATE CAT

C   D

L7
iSt
iVL
coSt
coVL

1 s

Fig. 2. Antidromic discharges recorded from the proximal stump of cut
dorsal root filaments may be modulated by exteroceptive stimul-
ations. (A) unit from L6 during fictive locomotion in the spinal
cat. The efferent locomotor activity shows clear alternating
flexor activity (iSarL, iSt) although, in this particular case,
the extensor activity (iSmA) was not clearly evident. The tonic
discharge of the unit is clearly independent of the locomotor discharges. (B) the discharge of the same unit is markedly modulated
by alternating flexion and extension of the contralateral hip.
Dots represent the beginning of flexion. (C) unit from L7 in the
non-paralyzed decorticate cat. Bursts of discharge are induced by
dorsiflexion (beginning marked by the dots) of the ipsilateral
foot. Electromyograms were recorded from the semitendinosus (St)
and vastus lateralis (VL) muscles in the ipsi- (i) and contralateral (co) hindlimb. (D) as the cat walked on the treadmill,
the unit discharged during the ipsilateral flexor burst (iSt).

rate during flexion and was silent during extension. During flexion of the
contralateral hip, the discharge frequency of the unit reached 50 Hz as
compared to 22 Hz when there was no manipulation of the hindlimb. Moreover, since the locomotor rhythm was not entrained by the manipulation of
the contralateral limb but the discharge of the cell was, it is improbable
that the modulation of the unit discharge would result from an indirect
action via the generator for locomotion. It is interesting that the discharge of the unit did follow closely rapid alternations of passive flexion
and extension (1.6 Hz in Figure 2B); such values fall within the natural
range of limb motion frequencies which are observed during locomotion of
intact cats (Halbertsma, 1983). Thus, one could speculate that during real
locomotion, peripheral input originating from the rhythmically flexing and
extending contralateral hip, could similarly modulate the polarization of
primary afferents.

It is noteworthy that exteroceptive stimulation over relatively wide
peripheral regions could induce or modulate antidromic firing of these
primary afferents. For example, not only was the discharge of the unit in
Figure 2B increased by flexion of the contralateral hip, but it was also
markedly decreased by mild pressure applied over the medial and anterior
aspect of the ipsilateral thigh. Other units were excited from both hindlimbs while yet other units had receptive areas restricted to the ipsilateral foot pads. In the non-spinalized decorticate preparation, some
antidromic unit discharges were even modulated by passive movement of the
ipsi and/or the controlateral forelimb.

Similarly, in the non-paralyzed decorticate cat at rest, manipulation of the hindlimbs could induce antidromic bursts of discharge in primary afferents such as shown in Figure 2C. As the ipsilateral foot was passively dorsiflexed (marked by a dot), the unit began to discharge. It stopped as the foot was ventroflexed back to its original position. When the cat was allowed to walk on a moving treadmill belt, the same unit showed clear bursts of discharge at the periodicity of the locomotor cycle (Figure 2D). Indeed, a burst of impulses was discharged during the period of activity of the ipsilateral flexor muscle, iSt, a time of the step cycle when there is active dorsiflexion at the ankle (Halbertsma, 1983). Therefore, it is possible that as the cat walks, the discharge of the unit may be triggered by some phasic input related to the active dorsiflexion of the ipsilateral foot.

It is justifiable to assume that the dorsal root discharges occur when depolarization of the afferent terminals is sufficient to initiate an antidromic action potential. The antidromic discharges may thus be regarded as giving an indication of the depolarization of single afferent terminals. The present results suggest that, during rhythmic movements, presynaptic actions on the primary afferent terminals may have two origins: a central and a peripheral one. During fictive locomotion, the spinal cord is deprived of any movement-related phasic input from the periphery. Still, rhythmic antidromic bursts of discharge occur in cut dorsal root filaments at fixed times during the locomotor cycle in both the decorticate and spinal preparation. This suggests that the central generator (CPG) for locomotion exerts phasic depolarizing actions on the primary afferent terminals. It remains to be determined, however, if it acts differentially with regards to different populations of primary afferents. In view of the presence of discharges in different phases of the locomotor cycle (Dubuc et al., 1986), it is probable that the primary afferent terminals may be subjected to differential effects. However, it is not yet determined if the discharges which occur in different phases of the step cycle may be attributed to differences in the modality and/or the receptive field of the afferent fibers.

It is noteworthy that the antidromic discharge of many other units (60%) was not modulated by the central rhythm. Most interestingly however, is the fact that some could either be induced or modulated by passive manipulations of the hindlimbs. Similarly, Matthews (1934) in his early work, has reported on the presence of antidromic action potentials in the dorsal roots which were modulated by manipulations of either hindlimbs or in some cases, by the forelimbs. Such discharges were classed as relayed discharges (Barron and Matthews, 1935). It is our belief that units such as the one illustrated in Figure 2 are of the same kind, and most certainly underscore the possibility that during locomotion, peripheral input may also exert important polarizing actions on the primary afferent terminals and that those actions may come from the same or even other moving limbs.

It is thus likely that during real locomotion, the presynaptic polarization which undoubtably occurs at the primary afferent terminals is a composite of phasic, and perhaps also tonic, inputs from the moving limbs with a central action by the CPG. Finally, from a functional standpoint, the interest of the present results centers on the fact that presynaptic actions might play very important roles in the modulation of some peripheral input during locomotion. For instance, it is not unlikely that the phasic modulation which occurs in some cutaneous reflex responses during locomotion (for review, see Rossignol and Drew, 1985) might be partly attributable to mechanisms acting at the level of the primary afferent terminals themselves. Furthermore, there are indications that the reflex modulation appears to depend both on central (Andersson et al., 1978) and peripheral (Grillner and Rossignol, 1978) effects as reported here for the polarizing actions on the primary afferent terminals.

Acknowledgments

This work was supported by a Group grant from the Canadian MRC. Thanks are due to Messrs S. Bergeron, G. Blanchette, R. Bouchoux, and D. Cyr, as well as to Miss J. Provencher for their technical contributions. J. -M. Cabelguen was supported by a fellowship from the France-Canada exchange program (CNRS-CNRC) as well as from the Centre de Recherche en Sciences Neurologiques de l'Université de Montréal.

REFERENCES

Andersson, O., Forssberg, H., Grillner, S., and Lindquist, M., 1978, Phasic gain control of the transmission in cutaneous reflex pathways to motoneurones during 'fictive' locomotion, Brain Res., 149:503-507.

Barron, D. H., and Matthews, B. H. C., 1935, Intermittent conduction in the spinal cord, J.Physiol.(Lond.), 85:73-103.

Bayev, K. V., and Kostyuk, P. G., 1982a, Primary afferent depolarization evoked by the activity of spinal scratching generator, Neurosci., 6:205-215.

Bayev, K. V., and Kostyuk, P. G., 1982b, Polarization of primary afferent terminals of lumbosacral cord elicited by the activity of spinal locomotor generator, Neurosci., 7:1401-1409.

Dubuc, R., Cabelguen, J. -M., and Rossignol, S., 1985, Rhythmic depolarizations of lumbo-sacral and cervical dorsal roots during fictive locomotion, Soc.Neurosci.Abstr., 11:881.

Dubuc, R., Cabelguen, J. -M., and Rossignol, S., 1986, Rhythmic antidromic discharges of single primary afferents recorded in cut dorsal root filaments during locomotion in the cat, Brain Res. (in press).

Eccles, J. C., Schmidt, R. F., and Willis, W. D., 1963, The mode of operation of the synaptic mechanism producing presynaptic inhibition, J.Neurophysiol., 26:523-538.

Grillner, S., and Rossignol, S., 1978, Contralateral reflex reversal controlled by limb position in the acute spinal cat injected with clonidine i.v., Brain Res., 144:411-414.

Halbertsma, J., 1983, The stride cycle in the cat: The modelling of locomotion by computerized analysis of automatic recordings, Act.Physiol.Scand., Suppl.521.

Matthews, B. H. C., 1934, Impulses leaving the spinal cord by dorsal nerve roots, J.Physiol.(Lond.), 81:29P-31P.

Perret, C., and Cabelguen, J. -M., 1980, Main characteristics of the hindlimb locomotor cycle in the decorticate cat with special reference to bifunctional muscles, Brain Res., 187:333-352.

Rossignol, S., and Drew, T., 1985, Interactions of segmental and suprasegmental inputs with the spinal pattern generator for locomotion, in: "Feedback and Motor Control," W. J. P. Barnes and M. H. Gladden, ed., Croom Helm Ltd., London (in press).

RESPONSES OF THE FORELIMB TO PERTURBATIONS APPLIED

DURING THE SWING PHASE OF THE STEP CYCLE

T. Drew* and S. Rossignol

Centre de Recherche en Sciences Neurologiques
Département de Physiologie, Faculté de Médicine
Université de Montréal, Montréal, Canada

The ability of an animal to walk in different environments requires
that it is capable of incorporating into the locomotor rhythm any unexpected conditions that might impede its progress. The characteristics of the
adaptive responses elicited by an unexpected afferent volley have been
previously studied in intact cats in which cutaneous afferents were excited
either with electrical stimulation of the skin of the hindpaw or with
mechanical stimulation of the distal hindlimb and have been described in a
number of recent articles (Abrahams et al., 1985; Duysens and Loeb, 1980;
Duysens and Stein, 1978; Duysens et al., 1980; Forssberg, 1979; Wand et
al., 1980). However, very few reports have appeared on the effects of
similar stimuli to the forelimbs (see however, Matsukawa et al., 1982; Drew
and Rossignol, 1985). This paper describes the responses of the forelimbs
to unexpected perturbations given during the swing phase of locomotion and
the way in which such responses are incorporated into the locomotor cycle.

Experiments were performed on 5 chronically implanted and unrestrained
cats walking on a treadmill. Under barbiturate anesthesia, pairs of insul-
ated stainless steel wires were sewn into the belly of selected muscles of
the shoulder, elbow and wrist for electromyographic (EMG) recordings. In
addition, pairs of stainless steel wires held in a polymer cuff were placed
around the superficial radial nerve (SRn) for stimulation of cutaneous
afferents from the distal forelimb. All the wires were led subcutaneously
to small multi-connector plugs cemented to the skull.

Electrical stimulation of the SRn (single pulses of 0.2 ms duration)
is expressed in multiples of the current needed to evoke a just detectable,
short latency excitatory response in the brachialis muscle during the swing
phase of locomotion. In a terminal experiment it was determined that this
threshold value was only slightly superior to the threshold for eliciting
the shortest latency compound action potential in the nerve. Stimuli of
1.5 to 3.0 X T were given during every third step cycle. The time of the
stimulation within the step cycle was controlled by a delay circuit triggered from the onset of EMG activity in the brachialis muscle. Ten to
twenty stimuli were given at each phase of the step cycle. The EMGs and

---

*Correspondence to: Dr T. Drew, Centre de Recherche en Sciences
Neurologiques, Département de Physiologie, Faculté de Médicine, Université
de Montréal, P.O. Box 6128, Station A, Montréal, Québec, Canada H3C 3J7.

stimulus artifact were digitized at 1 KHz and analyzed off-line using a PDP
11/34 computer. A quantitative measure of the size of the response was
determined by integrating the reflex response and subtracting from it the
integrated EMG of a corresponding segment taken from unstimulated control
cycles (see Drew and Rossignol, 1984 for details).

All experiments were recorded on a video tape using a shutter camera
(2 ms exposure time each 16.7 ms i.e., 60 fields/s). The movement of the
limb was reconstructed by digitizing the coordinates of small reflective
points placed on the skin over bony landmarks (see Rossignol and Drew,
1985).

Figure 1 shows such reconstructed movements for a control and a
typical perturbed step cycle. In the normal step the limb follows a smooth
trajectory and during swing the foot is brought forward at a height which
is only slightly above the treadmill surface (Figure 1A and C). Figure 1B
illustrates the movement of the forelimb when its progress is perturbed at
the beginning of swing by a hand held rod equipped with a microswitch. In
the brisk response that follows, the limb is drawn away from the obstacle
and raised above it by a shoulder flexion; during this time the elbow is
locked and there is a slight dorsiflexion of the wrist (see Rossignol and
Drew, 1985). Following these initial actions there is a resumption of

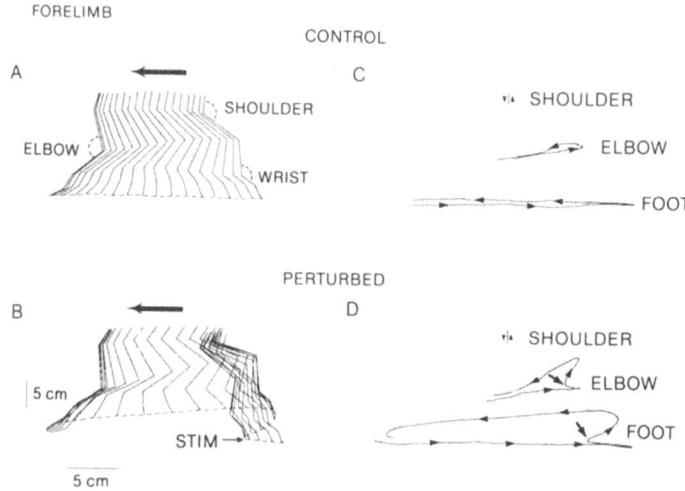

Fig. 1. Stick figures and limb trajectories of the forelimb reconstructed
from video records. Figures 1A and 1B show the movement of the
forelimb during swing in a control step cycle (A) and in a stimulated cycle (B). While walking on the treadmill the cat keeps a
constant position; however, for the purposes of these displays
each point on the leg has been separated from the identical point
on the preceding leg by a distance which is equal to the distance
moved by the foot. As a consequence the horizontal scale is twice
that of the vertical. The moment of mechanical stimulation is
indicated in (B) and the direction of travel is shown by the large
arrows above each figure. In (C) and (D) the trajectories of the
shoulder, elbow and foot are shown and are plotted with the
shoulder fixed in the sagittal plane. To facilitate the comparison with the stick figures of (A) and (B) these trajectories have
again been plotted with the horizontal scale twice that of the
vertical. The time of stimulation is indicated by the arrows in
(D).

elbow flexion, which together with a shoulder extension causes the limb to be brought forward over the obstacle; the wrist ventroflexes during this period to ensure that the foot does not recontact the obstacle.

The combined result of these angular changes on the trajectory of the foot and elbow can be more clearly seen in Figure 1D where it is evident that both the foot and the elbow are raised above their control positions due to the shoulder flexion. It should be noted that this is different from the situation in the hindlimb in which the foot is raised by knee flexion while the hip is locked (Wand et al., 1980; Rossignol and Drew, 1985).

Qualitatively similar results were seen with electrical stimulation of the SRn although the magnitude of the kinematic changes was always smaller than with the mechanical stimulation. This similarity, however, justified the use of electrical stimulation of the SRn to evaluate more rigorously the EMG responses underlying the kinematic changes.

Figure 2 shows an example of the averaged rectified responses recorded from representative muscles of the shoulder, elbow and wrist to electrical stimuli applied at approximately the same period of the step cycle as the mechanical stimulation shown in Figure 1. Both short and long latency

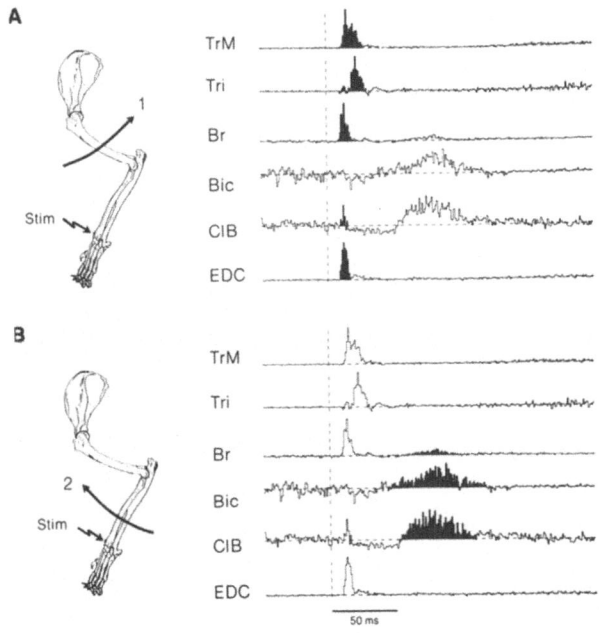

Fig. 2. Example of the early (A) and late (B) response evoked by an electrical stimulation of the SRn at a strength of 1.5 XT (150 μA). The averaged responses from 12 stimuli are displayed after subtraction of the activity during the control cycles. Consequently, all activity which is above the horizontal dotted line is a true excitation and all activity below the line is an inhibition. The regions most probably involved in the primary (A) and secondary (B) changes in limb trajectory have been shaded black. The arrows on the limbs to the left of the figure show the direction of the corresponding movement. Abbreviations: TrM, teres major; Tri, long head of triceps brachii; Br, brachialis; Bic, biceps brachii; ClB, cleidobrachialis; EDC, extensor digitorum communis.

responses were elicited by these stimuli. The short latency responses (Figure 2A) were coincident with the initial flexion of the shoulder, the locking of the elbow joint, and the extension of the wrist. The latency of these early excitatory responses lay within the range of 8-12 ms. In this example the initial response in Tri is small and is followed at a latency of 17 ms by a much larger response; however, in many cases both responses merge to form one large response with a latency of 9-12 ms. The cocontraction of elbow extensors (e.g., Tri) and elbow flexors (e.g., ClB and Br) is probably responsible for the locking of the elbow. A similar cocontraction has been observed in the extensor and flexor muscles of the ankle and has been suggested to be necessary for the locking of this joint while the knee is flexed above the obstacle (Wand et al., 1980). The teres major (TrM) undoubtedly contributes to the initial flexion at the shoulder while EDC is active during the wrist and digit dorsiflexion (physiological flexion).

Following the short latency responses there is a period of inhibition of the activity in biceps and cleicdobrachialis (and normally in brachialis) which is followed by a prolonged, long latency (40-80 ms) augmentation of the activity (Figure 2B). It is this hyperactivity which re-initiates the forward movement of the limb above and over the obstacle.

The response of the forelimb to a simple stimulus thus requires a coordinated activity of a number of flexor and extensor muscles of the shoulder, elbow and wrist. The nature of this response is such that the obstacle is quickly and smoothly negotiated and the normal locomotor pattern regained without causing any gross disturbance of the rhythm. This complex pattern, however, requires not only the enhancement of the amplitude of some muscles active during the swing phase of locomotion, but also the recruitment of other muscles such as triceps which are normally silent during this phase of the step cycle. This finding is all the more important since an identical stimulation when these extensor muscles are active in stance elicits no response (Drew and Rossignol, 1985). Thus the response in the extensors is obviously not due to the level of depolarization of motoneurones but must be mediated by internuncial relays whose excitability is high enough to activate motoneurones probably lying well beneath their firing threshold (see Cabelguen et al., 1981). This emphasizes the idea that effective compensatory responses of the limb during locomotion result from an active gain control of different reflex pathways. In this manner, already active muscles may be excited, inhibited or little changed and muscles which are inactive can be brought into action to lock a joint or to momentarily reverse the direction of the movement.

Acknowledgments

We would like to thank Messrs Bergeron, Blanchette and Bouchoux for their help in this project as well as Janyne Provencher who participated in both the experiments and the analysis. This work was supported by the Canadian MRC and by a grant from the FRSQ. T. Drew was supported by a FRSQ Scholarship.

REFERENCES

Abrahams, L. D., Marks, W. B., and Loeb, G. E., 1985, The distal hindlimb musculature of the cat. Cutaneous reflexes during locomotion, Exp.Brain Res., 58:594-603.

Cabelguen, J. -M., Orsal, D., Perret, C., and Zattara, M., 1981, Central pattern generation of forelimb and hindlimb locomotor activities in the cat, in: "Regulatory Functions of the CNS. Motion and Organisation Principles, Advances in Physiological Sciences, Vol. I," J. Szentagothai, M. Palkovits, and J. Hamori, eds., pp.199-211, Akedemiai Kiado, Budapest.

Drew, T., and Rossignol, S., 1984, Phase-dependent responses evoked in limb muscles by stimulation of the medullary reticular formation during locomotion in thalamic cats, J.Neurophysiol., 52:653-675.

Drew, T., and Rossingnol, S., 1985, Forelimb responses to cutaneous nerve stimulation during locomotion in intact cats, Brain Res., 329:323-328.

Duysens, J., and Loeb, G. E., 1980, Modulation of ipsi- and contralateral reflex responses in unrestrained walking cats, J.Neurophysiol., 44:1024-1037.

Duysens, J., Loeb, G. E., and Weston, B. J., 1980, Crossed flexor responses and their reversal in freely walking cats, Brain Res., 197:538-542.

Duysens, J., and Stein, R. B., 1978, Reflexes induced by nerve stimulation in walking cats with implanted cuff electrodes, Exp.Brain Res., 32:213-224.

Forssberg, H., 1979, Stumbling corrective reaction: a phase-dependent compensatory reaction during locomotion, 1979, J.Neurophysiol., 42:936-953.

Matsukawa, K., Kamei, H., Minoda, K., and Udo, M., 1982, Interlimb coordination in cat locomotion investigated with perturbation. I. Behavioural and electromyographic study on symmetric limbs of decerebrate and awake walking cats, Exp.Brain Res., 46:425-437.

Rossignol, S., and Drew, T., 1985, Interactions of segmental and suprasegmental inputs with the spinal pattern generator of locomotion, 1985, in: "Feedback and Motor Control," W. J. P. Barnes and M. H. Gladden, eds., Croom Helm Ltd., London (in press).

Wand, P., Prochazska, A., and Sontag, K. -H., 1980, Neuromuscular responses to gait perturbations in freely moving cats, Exp.Brain Res., 38:109-114.

COMPARATIVE ANALYSIS OF THE KINEMATICAL CHARACTERISTICS

OF MAN'S WALKING IN THE ONTOGENY

E. N. Artemjeva and V. V. Smolyaninov

Institute for Problems of Information Transmission
Academy of Sciences
Moscow, USSR

When a child learns to walk he learns something new. What is it? What kinematic changes of locomotion take place? Does the central nervous system acquire some new control programs in postnatal period or does the child learn to use the already available algorithms?

We tried to answer the question employing the method of analysis of the walking regularities applied before by Karpovich and Smolyaninov to describe the kinematics of walking of adults (Karpovich and Smolyaninov, 1975). The authors advanced a method of mathematical description of kinematic walking regularities employing invariants independent from speed, but taking into consideration both time and space characteristics of movements. This approach allowed to describe walking mathematically, as a clear-cut kinematic program, which is characterized by strict relations of such parameters as the period of step, the duration of the support and swing phases, the stride length etc., and the speed of movement. The program is characterized by the presence of two sinergies, which provide functional connections between independent parameters. They can be described as two invariants: the general - GI:

$$U = L_-/T_+ \tag{1}$$

and the complementary invariant - CI:

$$T_+ L = const \tag{2}$$

where $U_{(V)}$ put as a fractional-linear function in (1):

$$U(V) = (a_0 + a_1 V)/(1 + a_2 V).$$

In investigation of children's walking 20 normal and healthy subjects from 1.5 to 12 year's old took part. The data about age, stature etc., of each child are given in the Table 1. The instruction was to walk 'very slowly', than 'slightly faster', 'faster' and so on. All children were old enough to understand it. They made 6-25 transits, which were registrated by rapid cinephotography - 48 fr/s. Under magnification drawings were made from the film of the time-space movements of the extremity. For one leg the summary picture provides consecutive positions of the pelvis, knee-joint and projections on the ground of foot along axis - X. The drawings were used for measurements. Table 2 contains all analyzed parameters, method of their determination and their relations.

Table 1. Basic Data Referring to the Chosen Experimental Groups

No.	Group	Age (month) (year)	Subject	Sex	Stature (m)	Range of speeds (m/s)	Number of transits	Type of walk
1		8-9 m	A.Sh.	m	0.69	0.16-0.6	21	I
2	I	17 m	K.G.	f	0.75	0.5 -1.3	19	I
3		15 m	V.N.	f	0.74	0.6 -1.5	19	I
4		16 m	A.Sh.	m	0.82	0.4 -1.7	25	I
5		17 m	D.N.	m	0.83	0.5 -1.1	23	I
6		18 m	G.D.	m	1.00	0.3 -0.8	5	I
7	II	3-4 yr	S.S.	m	0.99	0.7 -1.3	9	II
8			S.K.	m	1.03	0.6 -1.9	10	II
9			O.S.	f	1.03	0.4 -1.5	13	II
10			N.D.	f	1.04	0.4 -3.0	17	I
11			V.I.	m	1.06	0.5 -1.7	10	I
12	III	4-5 yr	S.G.	m	1.06	0.6 -3.4	9	II
13			I.M.	m	1.13	0.9 -3.3	8	II
14	IV	8-9 yr	M.F.	m	1.21	0.9 -1.2	6	I
15			A.B.	m	1.35	0.3 -2.4	17	I
16			A.Uh	m	1.41	1.0 -3.7	13	II
17	V	11-12 yr	I.D.	f	1.41	1.0 -2.8	10	I
18			L.E.	f	1.43	0.7 -3.1	15	II
19			L.M.	f	1.46	0.7 -4.4	13	II
20			O.Ia	f	1.53	0.4 -2.5	10	I
21			I.Sh	f	1.54	1.1 -3.2	10	II

Basic relations of the kinematic parameters under study are presented on the Figure 1. Mean data on the different age groups is provided. These graphs led us to the conclusion, that the type of connections $T_{(V)}$, $T_{+(V)}$, $L_{(V)}$, $T_{+} L_{(V)}$ is similar for all the age groups under study, which means, that the approximations of these relations have similar analytical description. It is obvious, however, that the coefficients of the functions, describing these connections, must be different in different age groups. The greatest difference is observed between the adult and the youngest groups, but at the same time the difference between the children of 3-12 years is less substantial. Functioning of the complementary invariant $T_{+} L$ is crucial for the analysis of children's walking. Similarly with the tested adults, this quantity remains constant in the children's groups.

The parameter, characterizing the structure of the step cycle, that is quantity γ undergoes the most considerable transformations. Analysis of all the cases of the youngest age showed no relation between γ and speed. In the age of 3 to 12 year-olds with no noticeable correlation to stature, body proportions, range of the studied rates of the speed etc., two tendencies were observed with approximately similar frequencies: either γ remained constant while speed was growing (the 1 type of walking), or γ was growing while speed was growing, getting similar in it's functioning with the adult norm (the type II of the walking). The data obtained showed heterogeneity of the types of walking, which resulted in the reconsideration of the already described kinematic relations separately for each of the subgroups. The relations $T_{(V)}$, $T_{+(V)}$, $L_{(V)}$, $T_{+} L_{(V)}$ of the children groups, which we consider to be of the type II, were closer to the adult ones, than to the subgroup I. For this reason the type I of walking was called 'children' and the second one – 'adults'.

Table 2. The Analyzed Parameters and Relations

| Symbol | Quantity | How obtained | |
		measured	calculated
*V	walking speed	measured on the film or drawing	
T_+	time of swing	measured on the film or drawing	
T_-	time of support	measured on the film or drawing	
T	time of complete cycle of one leg		$T = T_+ + T_-$
γ	structure of cycle		$\gamma = T_+/T_-$
*L	stride length		$L = VT$
*L_-	stride length during support phase		$L_- = VT_-$
*U	speed during swing phase		$U = L_-/T_+$
GI	general invariant		**$F_1(U,V)$ = const
CI	complementary		***$F_2(L,T_+)$= const

*Relative characteristics of the given parameters, standartized by stature, were used.
**$F_1(U,V) = UV + a_1U + a_2V$.
***$F_2(L,T_+) = LT_+$.

Thus, the comparison of the kinematic parameters of the children's and adult walking showed, that all the basic relations, characteristic of this locomotion program become manifest already on the early stage of walking formation. Coincidence of the analytic forms of the step invariants can be interpreted as a sign of existence of universal program maintenance. The properties of the program, described by GI and CI can be traced from the age 1.5 which witnesses either to the very early formation, or to the 'genetic' derivation of the movement sinergy. Also data obtained through the analysis of locomotion kinematic characteristics of a child 8-9 months old speak in favor of the hypothesis of 'genetic' derivation of the basic structure of the walking program. Employing this material all the same relations can be traced at the same time the locomotion program is being perfected while a child is growing, which is connected with quantitive changes. The following fact should be paid attention to: variability of the kinematic walking characteristics in different age groups of children did not differ much (Figure 1). The observed ontogenetic stability of the weak relation between a step structure and walking speed, is obviously caused by some coordination transformations, solving, perhaps, the task of dynamic optimization, represented probably by the process of learning of 'adult' walking.

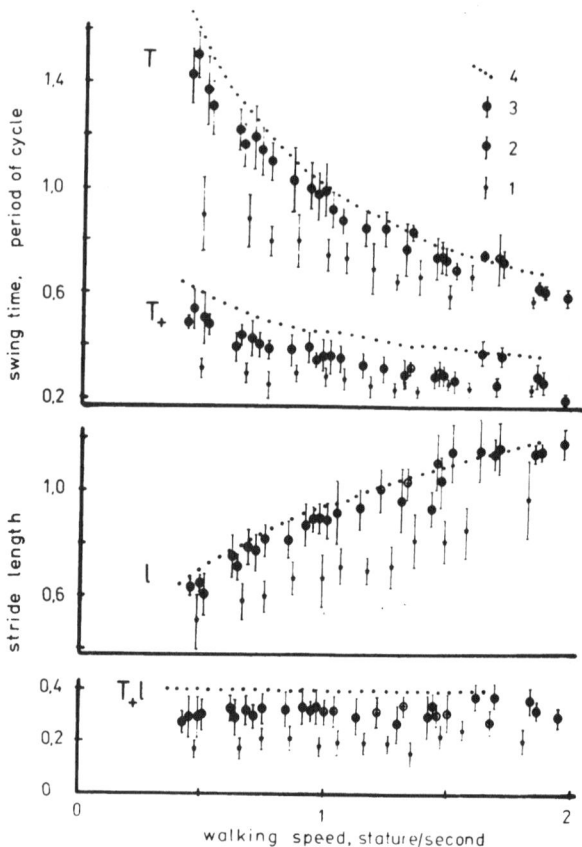

Fig. 1. Relations between basic kinematic parameters of walking for different age groups: (1) data for children of 1.5 years old; (2) 3-4 years; (3) 11-12 years and (4) adult subjects (last curve is reconstructed on the base of data provided by Karpovich and Smolyaninov, 1975). Mean values of the parameters are presented for each group. The parameters: V, L, L_+ are standartized by stature.

REFERENCES

Karpovich, A. L., and Smolyaninov, V. V., 1975, On the relations of kinematic characteristics of walking (in Russian), Physiologia cheloveka, I:167.

SECTION VI
MOTOR CONTROL MODELS

A MODEL FOR ONE-JOINT MOTOR CONTROL IN MAN

R. M. Abdusamatov, S. V. Adamovich, and A. G. Feldman

Institute of Information Transmission Problems
Academy of Sciences
Moscow, U.S.S.R.

It has been suggested that active movements may be the result of shifts in an equilibrium point (EP) specified by control signals derived from the brain (Feldman, 1974; Bizzi, 1980; Kelso and Holt, 1980). The aim of the present paper is to show that one of versions of the EP hypothesis (Feldman, 1974) may be used for explanation of kinematic and EMG patterns underlying the simplest one-joint movements. Figure 1 illustrates main concepts of the version of the EP hypothesis. In statics, the muscle is active if its actual length (x) exceeds a threshold length (λ). The recruitment of motor units and the muscle force increase with x-λ in the result of the tonic stretch reflex. The muscle force/length function for a given λ is called the invariant characteristic (IC; Figure 1A). The parameter λ is specified by the brain and may be considered an independent measure of central command descending to α and γ motoneurons. Instead of the variables x and λ we shall use now their angular equivalents: joint angle (ϕ) and threshold angle β (or β_1 for flexor muscles and β_2 for extensor ones; in some cases, e.g., in formulas (1) – (3) and Figure 1 flexor variables are used without the subscript). When flexor and extensor muscles of a single joint act together they yield a total IC (Figure 1B, dashed line). It intersects the displacement axis in a point which indicates an equilibrium position (r) of the system provided that the load is zero. It should be noted that $r = (\beta_1 + \beta_2)/2$ if the flexor and extensor ICs are of the same form as is supposed for the aim of simplicity. The r may be considered a central command which controls flexor-extensor coupled muscles as a coherent unit. Modifications of the r elicit a motion in the joint to the corresponding equilibrium position which is achieved if the system is damped enough, as is usually the case. Another coherent command, $c = (\beta_2 - \beta_1)/2$, specifies the magnitude of the angular zone in which the muscles are active simultaneously (Figure 1B). This command affects the slope (stiffness) of the total IC as is shown in Figure 1C.

In dynamics, not β but some other variable, $\beta*$, plays the role of the threshold for muscle activation. It has been argues (Feldman, 1974) that the $\beta*$ is a decreasing function of angular velocity ω. In linear approximation,

$$\beta* = \beta - \mu\omega \qquad (1)$$

where β is static flexor threshold and μ is a dynamic parameter (damping

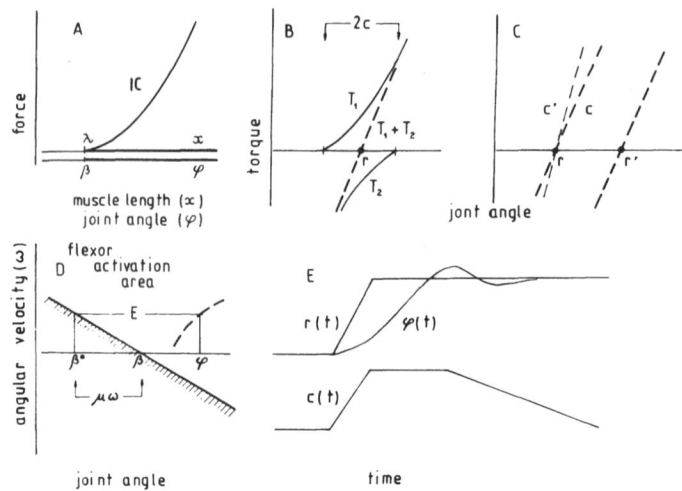

Fig. 1. Concepts of the equilibrium point hypothesis. (A) linear (λ) and angular (β) measures of a command parameter (activation threshold) for a muscle; invariant characteristic (IC). (B) total IC of a single joint (dashed) as a result of summation of flexor (T_1) and extensor (T_2) torques; coherent central commands r and c; equilibrium point (filled circle). (C) control of muscle stiffness and equilibrium position by c and r commands. (D) flexor activation area and its border (dashed) determined by the dependence of dynamic activation threshold (β^*) on angular velocity (ω); myoelectric activity (measurable by distance E) occurs when movement trajectory (e.g., as the dashed curve) penetrates into the area. (E) suggested temporal forms of central commands r and c for the simplest one joint movement $\phi(t)$ to a final position.

factor) which is suggested to be specified by γ dynamic motoneurons. Thus, the muscle is active if

$$\phi - \beta^* \geqslant 0 \qquad (2)$$

and the activity increases with $\phi - \beta^*$. Inequality (2) defines the dynamic muscle activation area (Figure 1D). It is naturally to assume that the variable $E = \phi - \beta^*$, with the reservation that $E = 0$ if $\phi - \beta^* < 0$, is a measure of flexor myoelectric activity. As (1) and (2) show, not only kinematic but also command variables affect muscle activity. Similarly, one may introduce a measure of extensor myoelectric activity.

The form of movement trajectories and EMG patterns essentially depend on the timing of the central commands (r, c, μ). Figure 1E shows the suggested temporal form of central commands r and c for rapid one-joint movements to various final positions without special instructions. The command r develops at a constant rate μ to a final value which determines a final equilibrium position of the joint. The μ is specified by the brain and essentially determines actual movement speed. The coactivation command c provides high stiffness of the system and, as a consequence, generation of meaningful forces needed for the execution of rapid movements. After the end of movement the support of high stiffness is unnecessary, and the coactivation command is gradually switching off.

The suggestion that rapid discrete movements are elicited by EP shifts at a constant rate makes it possible to represent every such a movement as a result of successive generation and superposition of identical movements having a smaller amplitude as is examplified in Figure 2A. Two natural trajectories (a and b) of the fastest movements in the elbow joint coincide during an initial time period (τ). There is also shown trajectory a shifted to the right by the time τ and 2τ and marked by a_1 and a_2. Computer summation of trajectories a, a_1 and a_2 gives rise to curves $a + a_1$ and $a + a_1 + a_2$ which approximate trajectory b much more than that a. The approximation could be absolute if the amplitude of the curve b were a multiple of that of the componential curve a (Adamovich et al., 1984). Acceleration curves may also be represented by a series of identical components (Figure 2B).

The above suggestion on the constant-velocity EP shifts allows us to associate the point of bifurcation of the curves a and b in Figure 2A with the completion of the EP shifts for the curve a. Thus, the τ is the duration of the EP shifts at a distance A equalled to the amplitude of curve a. The rate u of the shifts is given by $u = A/\tau = 560.4°/s$. For different subjects (n=5) the u was in the range of 500-700°/s.

For computer simulation of rapid one-joint movements the value $u = 600°/s$ was used. The coactivation command for simplicity was accepted to be constant. Muscle torque (T_i) in the model are given by

$$T_i = f_i(E_i) \qquad (3)$$

where E_i (i = 1, 2) are measures of flexor and extensor EMG activity; functions f_i describe the form of ICs. Dynamic properties of muscle torques are specified by the dependence of variables E_i on kinematic and command variables as is indicated above. However, it is obvious that some dynamic properties of muscles are not taken into account in (3).

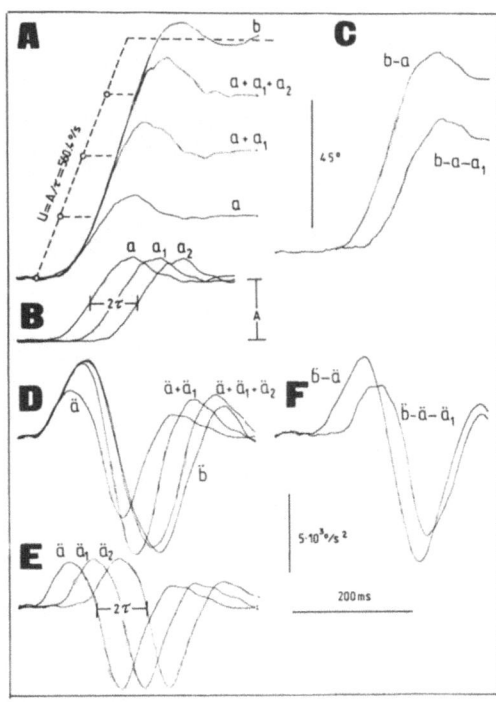

Fig. 2. Displacement (A - C) and acceleration (D - F) trajectories and their combinations during human movements about elbow. See text.

The above control organization in combination with the equation of motion for a single joint was numerically modelled. Because of simplifications concerning, in particular, muscle properties, the model illustrates only qualitatively the origin of kinematic and EMG patterns in the framework of the EP hypothesis but does not claim their exact correspondence to experimental data. Figure 3A shows an example of modelling of a rapid one-joint movement elicited by a central command r(t) which provides an uniform shift of the EP to a final position. The command gives rise to reciprocal flexor-extensor activity ('EMG') which is qualitatively consistent with the three-burst EMG pattern typical for natural fast one-joint movements. The pattern is sometimes observable in case of rapid isometric torque exertion (Gordon and Ghez, 1984). This result could indicate that the pattern is in the main programed centrally. On the other hand, during isometric condition an active muscle component contracts for the expense of extension of a passive, series elastic component. The inner muscle kinematics could still play a role in the determination of the isometric EMG pattern. The model must correspondingly be modified to take into account the two-component muscle structure. To a certain degree, one can imitate the series elastic component in the present model by introducing a stiff but still pliable load. Figure 3B shows that in such near-isometric conditions the model demonstrates 'EMG' bursts in response to a rapid monotonic command signal.

To summarize, the present experimental and theoretical results are consistent with the suggestion that the simplest rapid one-joint movements are executed by centrally specified constant-velocity shifts of the EP to a final position. The shifts give rise to EMG bursts without direct central programing of their time periods and amplitudes.

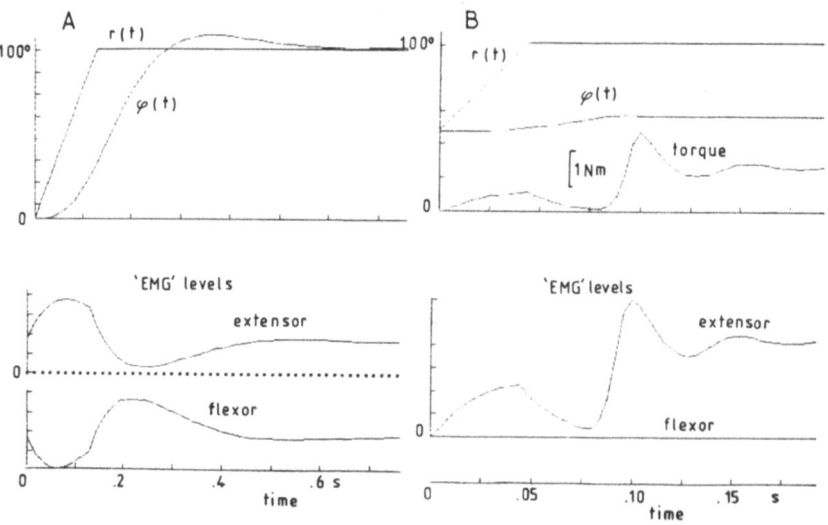

Fig. 3. Computer simulation of myoelectric patterns ("EMG" levels) and angular trajectories φ(t) of rapid one-joint movements against a zero load (A) and load increasing as an exponential function of the joint angle to constrain movement size (B). The kinematic and EMG patterns result from central commands r(t) which provide constant-velocity EP shifts to final positions.

REFERENCES

Adamovich, S. V., Burlachkova, N. I., and Feldman, A. G., 1984, On the
    central wave nature of time-angle trajectory formation in man,
    Biofizika, 29:122.
Bizzi, E., 1980, Central and peripheral mechanisms in motor control in:
    "Tutorials in Motor Behavior," G. E. Stelmach and J. Requin, eds.,
    North-Holland, Amsterdam.
Feldman, A. G., 1974, Control of the length of a muscle, Biophysics,
    19:776.
Gordon, J., and Ghez, C., 1984, EMG patterns in antagonist muscles during
    isometric condition in man: Relations to response dynamics,
    Exp.Brain Res., 55:167.
Kelso, J. A. S., and Holt, K. G., 1980, Exploring a vibratory system
    analysis of human movement production, J.Neurophysiol., 43:1183.

SYSTEM IDENTIFICATION IN MOTOR CONTROL:

TIME-VARYING TECHNIQUES

I. Hunter and R. Kearney

Biomedical Engineering Unit
McGill University
Montreal, Canada

INTRODUCTION

System identification techniques have found great applicability in the description of various dynamic aspects of the motor control system under time-invariant conditions. For example, the dynamic relation between small-amplitude angular displacements applied to the human ankle, and the resulting ankle torque at a constant mean torque, is well described by a linear, time-invariant dynamic-stiffness transfer function (Hunter and Kearney, 1982). The time-invariant dynamic-stiffness identification approach has also been successful in characterizing changes in the dynamic stiffness of the human ankle during slow (both large and small) changes in muscle activation levels (Hunter and Kearney, 1984a). However, during limb movement muscle forces and hence limb torques are often changing relatively rapidly, with the result that the mechanical dynamics can no longer be represented using time-invariant system identification techniques. Time-varying techniques are required.

Traditional approaches to the problem of characterizing a system (e.g., muscle) whose dynamics (e.g., muscle dynamic stiffness) are changing (e.g., during a muscle twitch) as a function of time (or some other domain) typically involve estimating the time-dependent parameters of some parametric linear dynamic model. The usual approach is to make some assumption about the system order and to use one of the recent recursive identification techniques (see Ljung and Soderstrom, 1983) to estimate the parameter trajectories.

In many areas of the life sciences, however, assumptions about the system order, and even whether or not the system is linear, are difficult to make. A more useful nonparametric approach would be to make only some assumption about the form of the system (e.g., linear, Hammerstein nonlinear, etc.) and to leave open the question of model order. However general, readily usable, nonparametric approaches to the identification of time-varying linear of nonlinear systems do not exist. We have developed a technique for the identification of time-varying linear or nonlinear systems which can be applied in those special circumstances (such as in muscle research) where the time-variation can be repeated.

TIME-VARYING IDENTIFICATION TECHNIQUE

The technique is derived from a highly novel approach to time-varying system identification which was independently developed by two groups (Lawrence and Dawson, 1977; Soechting, Dufresne and Lacquaniti, 1981). We have extended the technique to enable it to be used in our research on isolated muscle fiber mechanics and the dynamics of the human neuromuscular system. The method has also been implemented in NEXUS, a computer language for systems and signal analysis (Hunter and Kearney, 1984b). The following description of the technique is taken from Hunter and Kearney (1985).

Consider an input to a time-invariant dynamic linear system consisting of a 127 sample pseudo-random binary sequence (PRBS) (see Eykhoff, 1974). If the input is repeated 127 times then the dynamics of the system can be determined from each of the 127 127-length input and output data sets. However there is another way to determine the dynamics which involves firstly constructing 127 new data sets from the old 127 data sets. Each new data set is obtained by taking 1 sample from each of the old data sets such that the first sample in the n-th new set is the n-th sample of the first old set, the second sample in the n-th new set is the (n+1)-th sample from the second old set, and so on. Thus the idea is to construct a new data set by taking samples from across an ensemble of similar data sets. This is a trivial example because in such a time-invariant situation there would be no reason to go to the extra trouble in order to identify the system dynamics.

However the technique becomes immensely powerful when the dynamics of a system must be obtained under time-varying conditions (i.e., where the dynamics are changing). There is one crucial condition to be met before the technique can be applied. It must be possible to arrange for repetitions of the time-variation or transient (e.g., muscle twitch) to occur at different times with respect to the start of the input. Indeed these times must be arranged so that they occur at an increment in time further into the input sequence each time the input sequence is repeated. If this is achieved then an input and output data set can be constructed for each increment throughout the time-variation which is relatively unaffected by the time-variation. Each of these cross-ensemble input-output data sets may then be analyzed using time-invariant techniques. For example if a linear dynamic representation of the 'instantaneous' dynamics is desired then the impulse response function might be determined. The change in the system throughout the time-variation would then be represented by a surface of impulse response functions.

APPLICATION TO SIMULATED SYSTEM

Consider the second-order underdamped low-pass system defined in the s-domain as

$$H(s) = \frac{G \, \omega_n^2}{s^2 + 2\zeta\omega_n s + \omega_n^2}$$

where

$H(s)$ is the system transfer function,

ζ is the damping parameter,

ω_n is the natural frequency, and

G is the static gain.

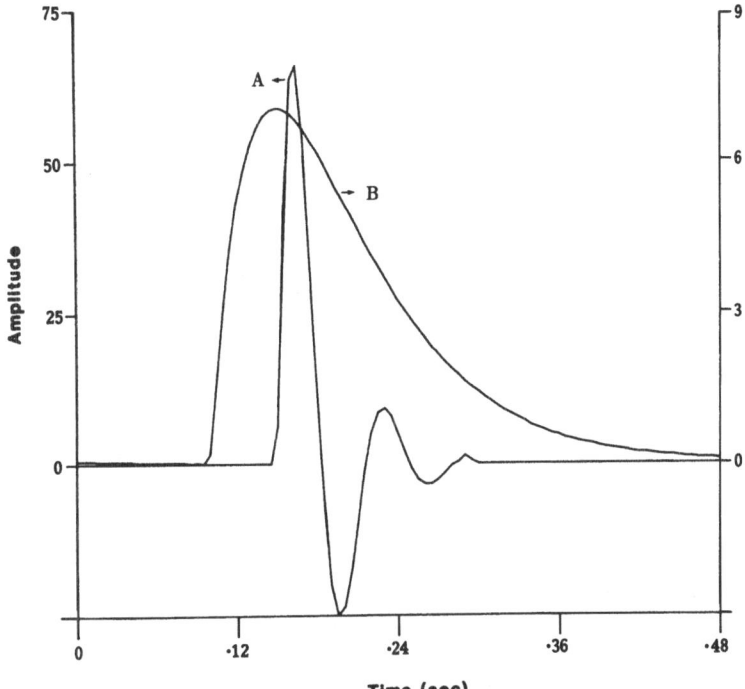

Fig. 1. (A) the simulated system impulse response function, $h(\tau)$; (b) the variation in the parameter, G, of the simulated system with time.

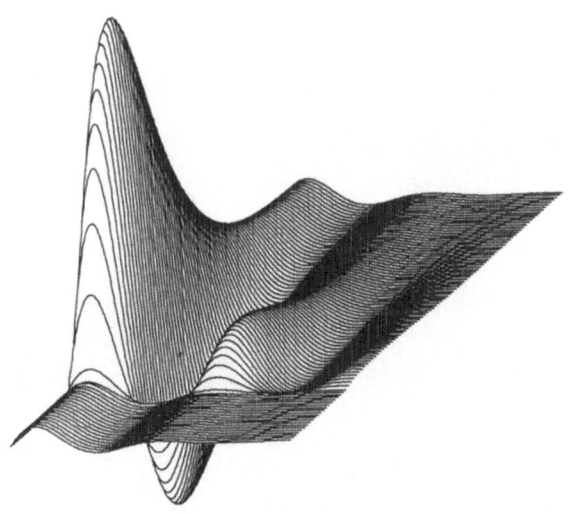

Fig. 2. The surface of impulse response functions which define the way in which the simulated system changes throughout the time-variation.

Figure 1 curve A is the inverse Laplace transform of $H(s)$, namely the system impulse response function, $H(\tau)$, when $\zeta = .3$, $\omega_n = 2\pi$ rads/sec and G assumes some arbitrary value. Figure 1 curve B specifies the variation of G with time. The gain, G, changes smoothly but rapidly through time from near zero to a maximum to near zero again. If the time variation of G was

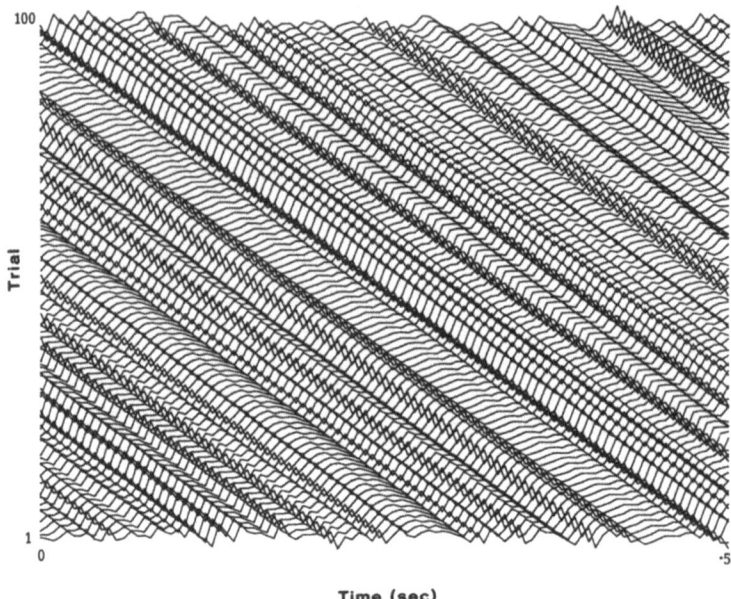

Fig. 3. The ensemble of inputs used in the time-varying identification
technique.

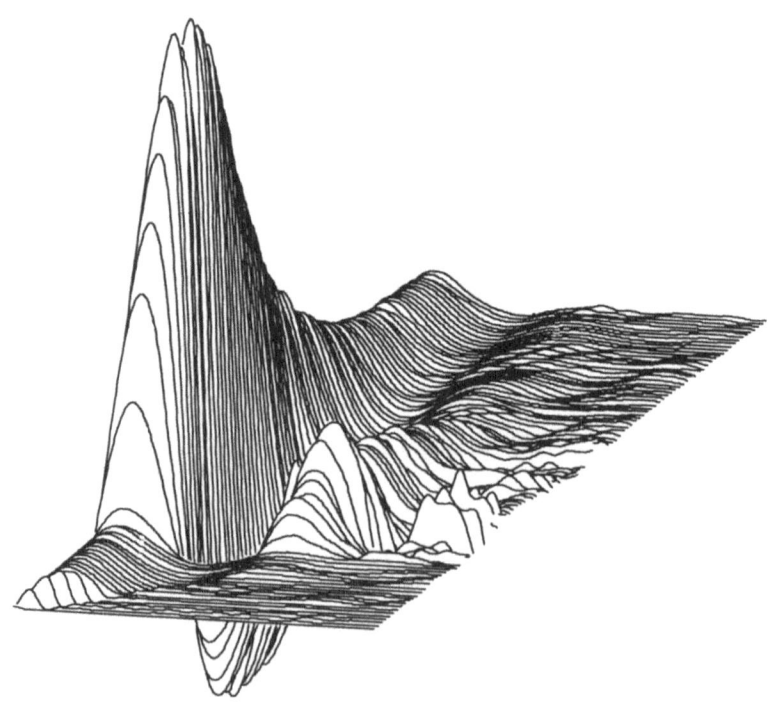

Fig. 4. The surface of estimated impulse response functions characterizing
the way in which the simulated system changes throughout the
time-variation.

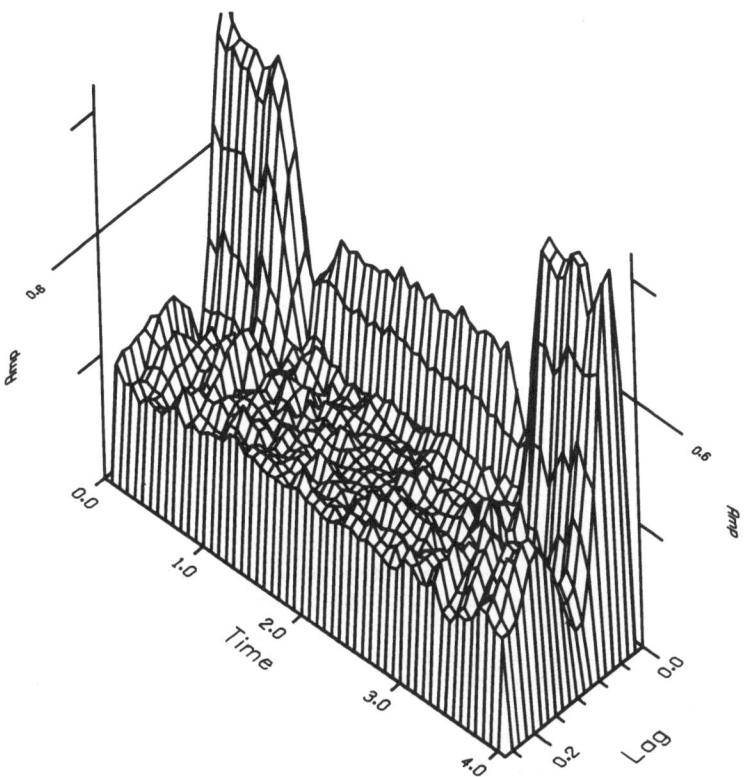

Fig. 5. A compliance impulse response surface estimated from the ensemble of input-output data obtained from one subject.

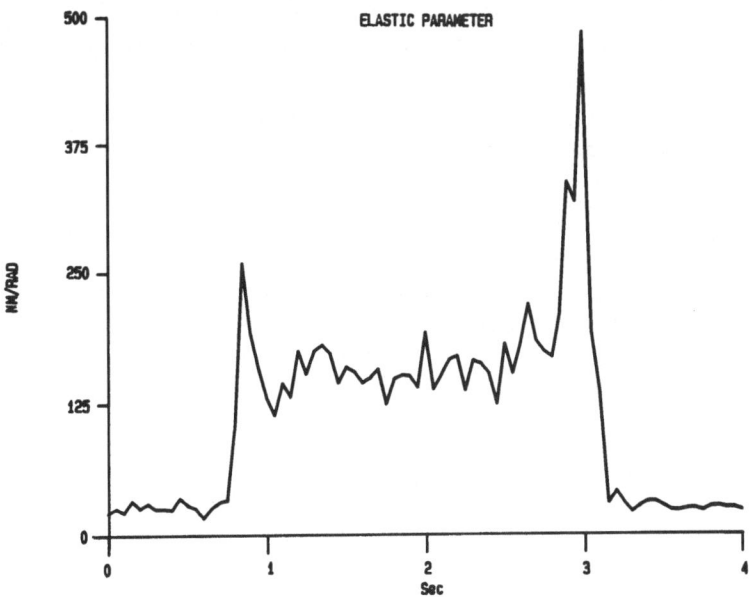

Fig. 6. The changes in elastic stiffness throughout the contraction.

slow compared with the during of the impulse response then time-invariant identification techniques could be used. However in the example the duration of h(τ) is of the same order as that of the time-variation. Time-varying identification techniques must be used here as time-invariant identification methods fail utterly under these conditions. Figure 2 shows the surface of impulse response functions which define the way in which the system changes throughout the time-variation.

The problem is to estimate this surface by performing experiments on the system. As specified by the time-varying identification method proposed the system is repeatedly perturbed by a stochastic input which is shifted by an increment with respect to the initiation of the time-variation on each successive trial. The ensemble of inputs used are shown in Figure 3. The results obtained by applying the time-varying identification technique to the system are shown in Figure 4. Comparison of the two surfaces (Figures 2 and 4) clearly shows the power of the technique.

APPLICATION TO NEUROMUSCULAR SYSTEM

We now illustrate the use of the time-varying identification method in an experiment (Kearney and Hunter, 1985) in which we have used it to measure changes in the dynamic stiffness (or its dynamic inverse, compliance) of the human ankle during rapid changes in mean muscle force levels of the ankle plantarflexors (triceps surae) and dorsiflexors (tibialis anterior). Subjects changed repeatedly from one mean ankle torque level to another mean torque level as fast as possible, while their ankles were perturbed by a small stochastic angular displacement. The perturbations were delivered by an electro-hydraulic ankle actuator which had a frequency response to 50 Hz. The onset of the contraction with respect to the stochastic input was changed by an 5 msec increment on each successive trial.

Figure 5 shows a compliance impulse response surface estimated from the ensemble of input-output data obtained from one subject. The decreased compliance resulting from the contraction is evident in the figure. The changes in elastic stiffness (estimated by fitting a second-order model to each impulse response function) throughout the contraction are shown in Figure 6. Of particular interest is the augmented elastic stiffness evident during the onset and termination of the contraction.

The time-varying identification method should prove of use in many other areas of motor control research.

Acknowledgments

Supported by grants from the Medical Research Council of Canada and the Natural Sciences and Engineering Research Council of Canada.

REFERENCES

Eykhoff, P., 1974, "System Identification: Parameter and State Estimation," Wiley, London.

Hunter, I. W., and Kearney, R. E., 1982, Dynamics of human ankle stiffness: variation with mean ankle torque, J.Biomech., 15:747.

Hunter, I. W., and Kearney, R. E., 1984a, Invariance of ankle dynamic stiffness during fatiguing muscle contractions, J.Biomech., 16:985.

Hunter, I. W., and Kearney, R. E., 1984b, NEXUS: A computer language for physiological systems and signal analysis, Comput.Biol.Med., 14:385.

Hunter, I. W., and Kearney, R. E., 1985, A technique for the identification of time-varying system dynamics, Proc.11th Can.Med.Biol.Engin.Conf., p.3.

Kearney, R. E., and Hunter, I. W., 1985, Identification of neuromuscular dynamics of the human ankle during time-varying contractions, Soc.Neurosci.Abstr., 11:214.

Lawrence, P. J., and Dawson, R. D., 1977, Identification of periodic non-stationary antenna stabilisation control systems by cross-correlation techniques, IEEE Proc., 124:797.

Ljung, L., and Soderstrom, T., 1983, "Theory and Practice of Recursive Identification," MIT Press, Cambridge.

Soechting, J. F., Dufresne, J. R., and Lacquaniti, F., 1981, Time-varying properties of myotatic response in man during some simple motor tasks, J.Neurophysiol., 46:1226.

WORKSPACE EFFECT IN ARM MOVEMENT KINEMATICS

DERIVED BY JOINT INTERPOLATION

J. M. Hollerbach, S. P. Moore, and C. G. Atkeson

Massachusetts Institute of Technology
Center for Biological Information Processing and
Artificial Intelligence Laboratory, Massachusetts, U.S.A.

For unrestrained vertical arm movements measured with a Selspot system, it had been previously found that significantly curved endpoint trajectories occur in certain regions of the workspace, but that in other regions the trajectories are approximately straight (Atkeson and Hollerbach, 1985). Straight-line trajectories in hand space have been taken as evidence for movement planning in hand coordinates (Morasso, 1981), but the curved trajectories are a relatively new observation that were unexplained.

When trajectories are specified as straight lines in joint space, curved Cartesian trajectories could in principle result (Hollerbach and Atkeson, 1985). This strategy is known in robotics as joint interpolation (Brady et al., 1982). We have studied whether the experimentally observed curved trajectories can be explained in this way, or whether some other planning strategy is in effect. Our results show that the curved movements can be explained by a joint interpolation strategy. Moreover, when the definition of joint interpolation is generalized to allow a staggering in relative joint motion onset, the observed straight endpoint trajectories could be generated. Thus the strategy of staggered joint interpolation provides a unifying explanation for both straight and curved movements, and we conclude all trajectories could be planned in terms of joint coordinates.

INTRODUCTION

The search for invariances or regularities in human arm movements involves finding a set of variables that most concisely describes the experimental trajectories. This search is motivated first by identifying the planning variables that the motor control system may be using in the movement, and second by inferring the limitations that may exist in trajectory formation ability. That the simplest description of movement is evidence for planning in terms of this description's variables is a research strategy founded in the application of Occam's razor. In the present context, this strategy can also be considered a heuristic application of Bernstein's principle of equal simplicity (Bernstein, p.52):

"If we are concerned with any given system, the structure of which is unknown to us but whose operation we may observe under a variety of conditions, then by a comparison of the changes in the variable S (speed, accuracy, variation, etc.) encountered as a function of each of the variables in the conditions, we may come to determinate conclusions as to the structure of the system which are unattainable by direct means".

In examining drawing movements, Bernstein concluded that the invariant topology in different regions of the workspace suggested a representation of movement in terms of external space variables instead of joint variables or muscle variables. Morasso (1981) reached a similar conclusion in the study of two-joint arm movements in a horizontal plane measured by a planar pantograph. Regardless of the location of the endpoints, the trajectory was always found to approximate a straight line. Flash and Hogan (1985) described movement in terms of minimum jerk of the endpoint variables. Their model was capable of explaining the kinematic features of induced curved movements in the same experimental setup as that of Morasso (Abend, Bizzi, and Morasso, 1982). It has also been argued from a teleological standpoint that environmentally constrained motions imply a planning of movement in terms of endpoint variables (Hildreth and Hollerbach, 1986).

Planning of movement in terms of joint variables has also been advocated. Kots and Syrovegin (1966) described straight lines in joint space during coordinated flexion of the elbow with a roll motion along the forearm. Soechting and Lacquaniti (1981) showed evidence that in the deceleratory phase in an outward reaching movement in a vertical plane the ratio of elbow joint velocity to shoulder joint velocity tended towards a constant. This strategy was shown equivalent to joint interpolation in (Hollerbach and Atkeson, 1985). More recently, Soechting, Lacquaniti, and Terzuolo (1985) investigated figural movements with the arm in various movement planes, and found characteristic distortions arising from stereotypical joint variable relationships. The controlled joint variables were initially identified through a psychophysical investigation (Soechting and Ross, 1984).

The inference of planning variables from experimental measurements is a difficult task fraught with pitfalls. Planar two-joint kinematics has some surprising subtleties that defeat our intuitions. Hollerbach and Atkeson (1985) demonstrated a peculiar property of two-joint arm movement when approaching the workspace boundary. The joint rate ratio at the boundary is a constant dependent only on the link lengths and not on the trajectory that teached the boundary. Thus the tendency towards a constant joint rate ratio seen by Soechting and Lacquaniti (1981) is an artifact and is not evidence for joint variable planning. It is shown in the present paper that staggered joint interpolation can generate nearly straight lines in certain parts of the workspace. Thus endpoint straight lines cannot be taken by themselves as evidence for endpoint variable planning. Other issues include the variety of movements examined, the resolution of measurement, and the extraction of the metric aspects of a trajectory to fit a model. Finally, it must always be kept in mind that one's a priori models do not span the space of possible planning variables or strategies.

METHODS

Kinematic features of trajectories during point-to-point reaching movements were measured with a Selspot I system. LED targets under computer control were set in a sagittal plane, and were arranged to form four target pairs: a horizontal pair, a vertical pair, and two diagonaling pairs (Figure 1). Subjects were required to move from a start target to a goal target at various speeds and holding different weights. No spatiotemporal accuracy constraints were placed on the movement, which terminated when the pointing finger was roughly in front of the target LED without touching.

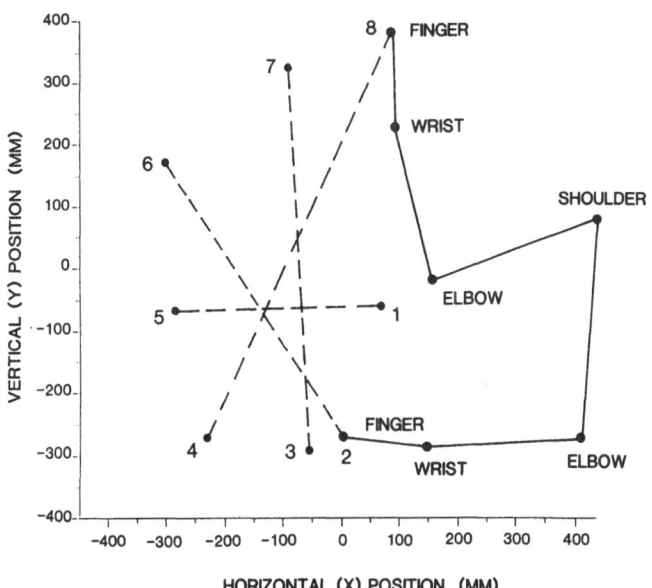

Fig. 1. Planar projection of the arm and the LED targets in the sagittal target plane. Four pairs of targets, numbered consecutively in the clockwise direction, defined four movement directions.

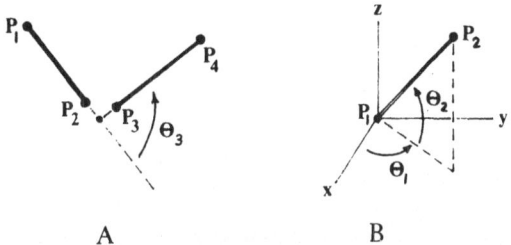

Fig. 2. (A) An upper arm bar with LEDs attached at the ends P_1P_2 and a forearm bar with LEDs at P_3P_4 The elbow angle θ_3 was calculated as the relative exterior angle between the bars. (B) Shoulder angles corresponding to a yaw motion θ_1 followed by a pitch motion θ_2 were calculated from the first bar.

Five infrared LEDs were attached to a subject's arm for tracking by the Selspot system. One was placed on the fingertip, and the other four were placed on the ends of two bars attached to the forearm and upper arm, respectively. These paired LEDs corresponded roughly to the position of the wrist, elbow, and shoulder. Three-dimensional coordinates of these LEDs as a function of time were calculated by triangulation, at a sampling rate of 315 Hz.

Joint angles for the shoulder and elbow were calculated from the four LEDs attached to bars, indicated by the points P_1 and P_2 for the upper arm bar and P_3 and P_4 for the forearm bar (Figure 2). The shoulder angles were defined in terms of a horizontal yaw motion θ_1 followed by a vertical pitch motion θ_2; a third shoulder roll motion was not calculated. These shoulder angles correspond to the psychophysical variables determined by Soechting and Ross (1984). The calculation of more than one shoulder angle was necessary because the elbow point typically came out of the vertical target plane, even though the fingertip and wrist usually stayed within the plane. The elbow angle θ_3 was calculated as the relative angle to the upper arm, in contrast to the absolute forearm angle suggested in (Soechting and Ross, 1984). From Figure 2,

$$\theta_1 = \tan^{-1}\left(\frac{y_2-y_1}{x_2-x_1}\right)$$

$$\theta_2 = \tan^{-1}\left(\frac{z_2}{\sqrt{(x_2-x_1)^2+(y_2-y_1)^2}}\right) \qquad (1)$$

$$\theta_3 = \tan^{-1}\left(\frac{v_1 \times v_2}{v_1 v_2}\right)$$

where $P_i = (x_i, y_i, z_i)$, $v_1 = P_2 - P_1$ and $v_2 = P_4 - P_3$. In the plots of shoulder angle versus elbow angle, the pitch shoulder angle θ_2 was used. More details of the experimental procedure may be found in (Atkeson and Hollerbach, 1985).

RESULTS

Typical results for the trajectories are shown in Figure 3. Plots 3A-3D represent trajectories projected into the sagittal target plane for the five tracked LEDs. Plots 3E-EH represent joint angle plots of shoulder versus elbow. It had been found in these experiments that the path and the tangential velocity profile were invariant across speed changes and hand-held loads for all subjects.

The horizontal 3A and outward and upward diagonal movements 3B were always straight in all subjects tested, while the vertical 3C and the inward and upward diagonal movements 3D were always curved. With regard to the two curved movements 3C and 3D, the corresponding joint angle plots 3G and 3H indicate straight lines in joint space. In the joint angle plot 3G for the vertical movement, the elbow was essentially frozen. Thus the movement is curved because it was produced almost exclusively by single-joint shoulder flexion, and hence is trivially an incidence of joint interpolation. For the joint angle plot 3H of the inward and upward diagonal movement, the joint angle plot is clearly a straight line in joint space. In this case, both joints were simultaneously active. Thus the initial supposition that the curved trajectories may be resulting from a strategy of joint interpolation was correct.

Rather than accept a hypothesis that two different coordination strategies are in effect in different parts of the workspace, the two straight trajectories in hand space were examined more closely for a possible alternative explanation. The horizontal movements 3A actually represent a straight line intersecting the shoulder joint, a known degenerate situation in which the joint-space trajectory 3E is also straight (Hollerbach and Flash, 1982). Thus it is a matter of viewpoint whether the horizontal trajectories are planned in hand or joint coordinates, and these trajectories when interpreted as joint interpolation are consistent with the two curved trajectories.

This leaves 3B as the only trajectory not explainable by joint inter-polation, since the joint angle plot 3F is clearly not straight. Nevertheless, if the definition of joint interpolation is generalized slightly to allow one joint to be staggered in onset relative to the other and for its time profile to be scaled uniformly, then trajectory 3B can be generated

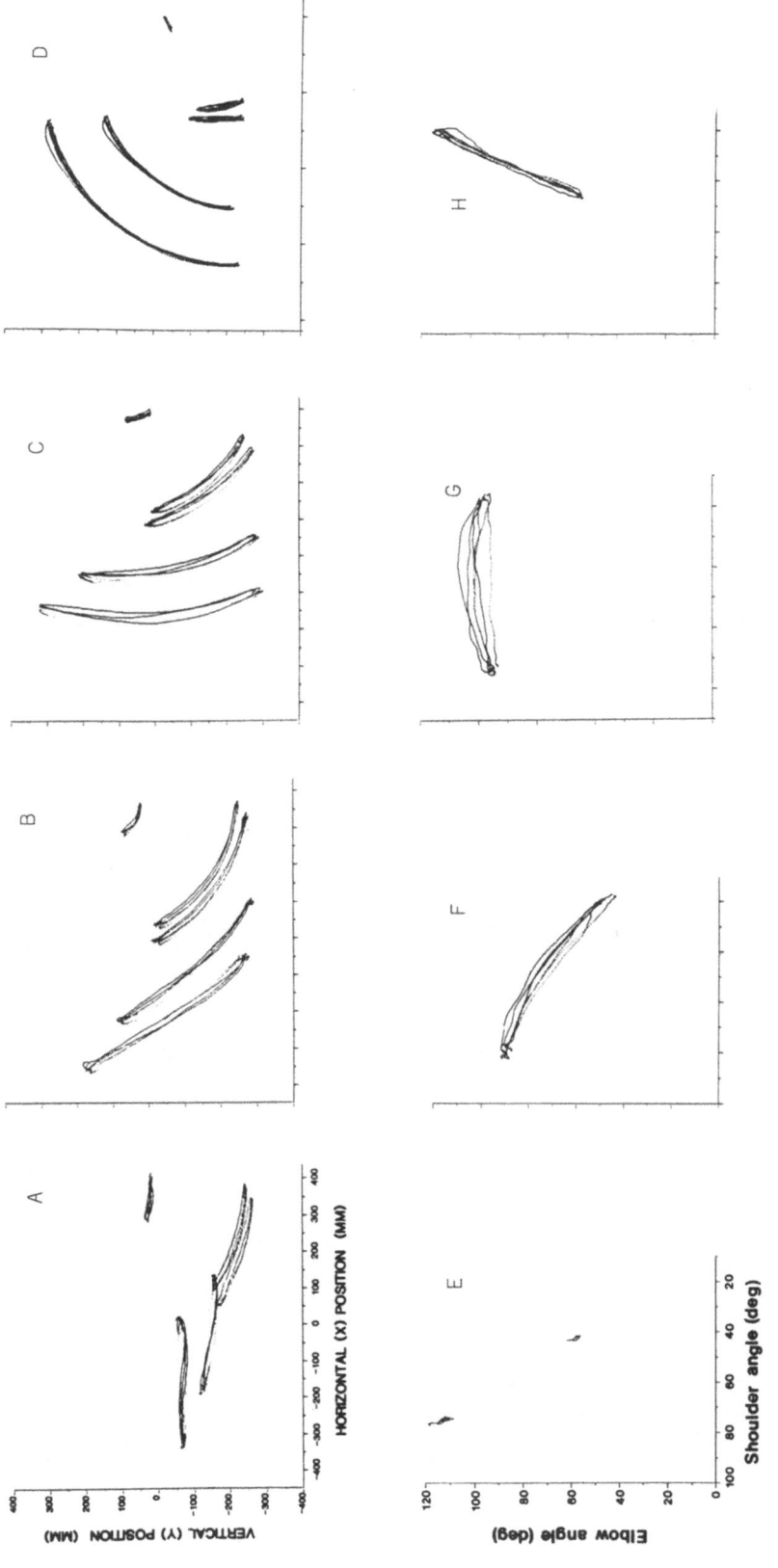

Fig. 3. (A)-(D) LED trajectories in the sagittal target plane for the four experimental movements. In each plot the traces for each of the five LEDs attached to the arm as shown. Six movements are superimposed in each panel, three in one direction and three in the reverse direction. Except for (A), the upward movements are indicated by dotted lines, where the dots are equally spaced in time, and the downward movements are indicated by solid lines. In (A) the outward movements are indicated by dotted lines. (E)-(H) Joint angle plots of shoulder pitch angle θ_2 versus elbow angle θ_3 corresponding to plots (A)-(D) respectively.

and all trajectories are consistent with a strategy of joint variable planning. Under the normal definition of joint interpolation, each joint has the same tangential velocity profile scaled by the distance it must move through:

$$\theta_2(t) = f(t)\Delta\theta_2$$

$$\theta_3(t) = f(t)\Delta\theta_3 \tag{2}$$

where $f(t)$ is the normalized velocity time profile, $\Delta\theta_i = \theta_i(t_f) - \theta_i(0)$, and t_f is the movement duration. Thus the joints execute in lockstep the same velocity profile, starting and stopping together.

Now suppose the onset of joint 3 movement is staggered an amount δ relative to joint 2, and that the time profile $f(t)$ is scaled by a factor c. Then

$$\theta_2(t) = f(t)\Delta\theta_2$$

$$\theta_3(t) = f(ct + \delta)\Delta\theta_3 \tag{3}$$

The same time profile is kept, but it is merely shifted relative to the joint 2 time profile and uniformly expanded or compressed. The scaling is needed so that joint 3 can end at the same time as joint 2 if its start is different, or joint 3 can start at the same time as joint 2 if its finish is different. Given that one of these two conditions holds, this strategy has only one free variable δ since the other can be determined by $c = 1 - \delta/t_f$.

Simulation demonstrates the capability of staggered joint interpolation to explain the features of trajectory 3B. In Figure 4, trajectories have been generated by modeling a subject's arm lengths and using the beginning and final joint angles determined from the data. The solid line in 4B is the theoretical straight line in Cartesian space, and the solid line in 4A is the theoretical shoulder versus joint angle plot corresponding to it. The straight dotted line in 4A corresponds to a strategy of simple joint interpolation, which generates the outer curved trajectory

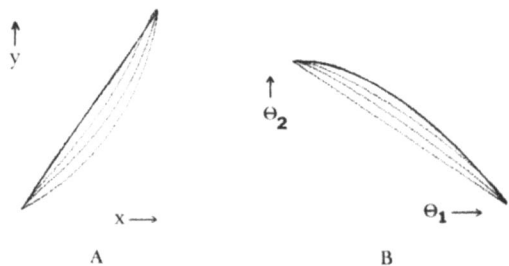

Fig. 4. Simulation of the movement corresponding to Figure 3D. In (A) the endpoint coordinates are plotted for a theoretical straight line trajectory (solid line) and for various staggered joint interpolations (dotted lines). In (B) the plot of shoulder versus elbow angle shows the theoretical curve (solid line) corresponding to an exact straight endpoint trajectory. Simple joint interpolation is shown in (B) by the straight dotted line, which generates the outer curve in (A). Increased staggering of relative joint onset produces a sequence of curves that approaches the theoretical straight-line motion.

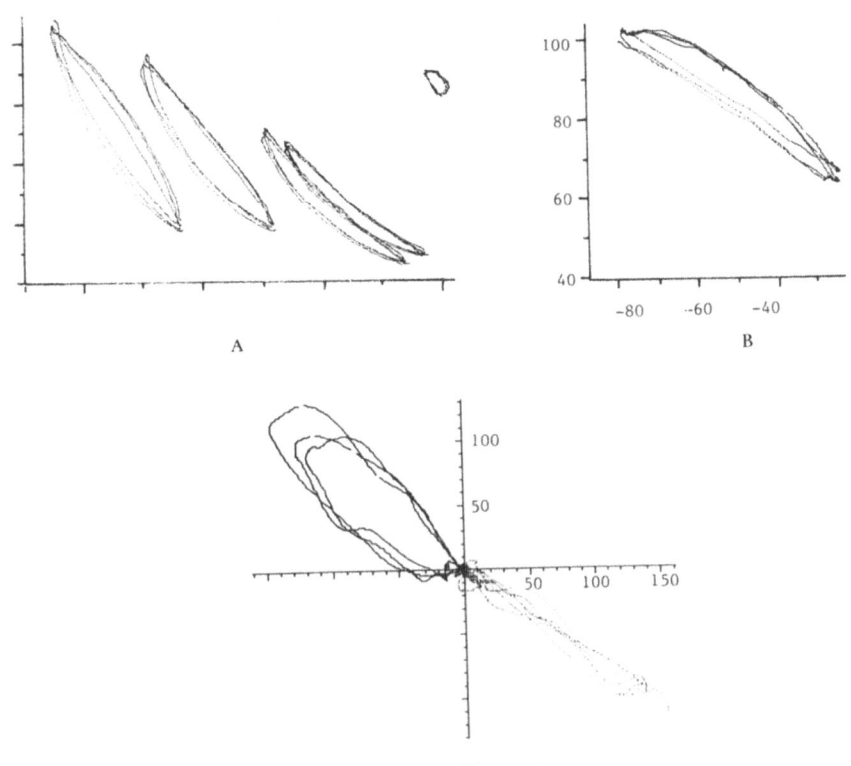

Fig. 5. (A) An outward and upward diagonal movement for a different
subject shows a trajectory difference depending on movement
direction. (B) The joint angle plot. The units are degrees.
(C) The plot of shoulder joint velocity versus elbow joint
velocity, in deg/sec.

in 4B. As the elbow is increasingly staggered in onset relative to the
shoulder, a sequence of curved lines approaches the theoretical solid lines
until they are practically indistinguishable.

In the plot of shoulder joint velocity versus elbow joint velocity
corresponding to trajectory 3B, an offset can barely be discerned as
periods of near-zero shoulder movement. Simulation shows that the
curvature of the trajectory is quite sensitive to even small offsets.
Other trajectories provided clearer evidence for staggered joint interpolation. A movement similar to 3B for a different subject is shown in
Figure 5A. This movement is typical of some trajectories where there were
differences between the two directions. The joint angle plot in 5B shows
that the outward direction was generated by simple joint interpolation, but
that the inward direction corresponded to a more complex joint angle trajectory. The plot of shoulder joint velocity versus elbow joint velocity
in 5C clearly shows a staggering of the elbow joint relative to the
shoulder joint for this inward movement. Hence this subject evidently used
simple joint interpolation in one direction, and staggered joint interpolation in the other.

A final example is one of the more drastic in demonstrating joint
offsets. The trajectory in Figure 6A is similar to that in 3D, but for a
different subject. The joint velocity plot in 6C shows a large decoupling

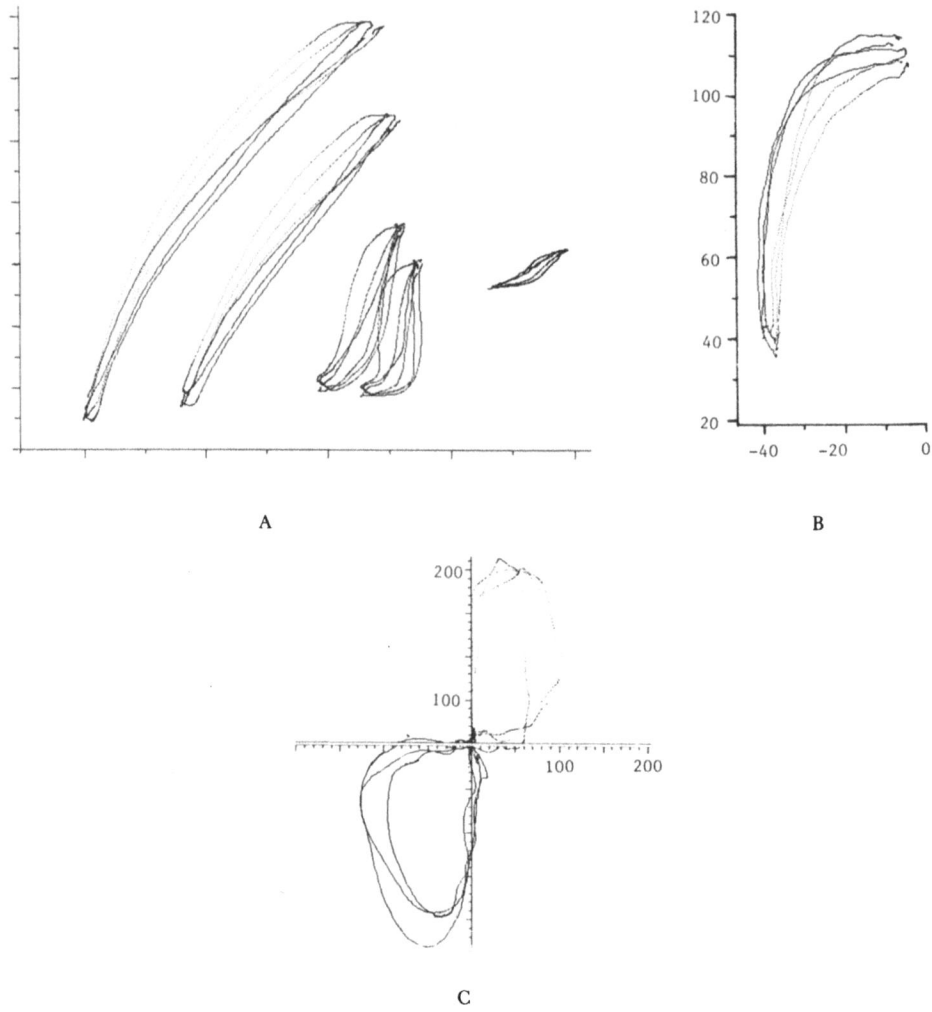

Fig. 6. (A) An inward and upward diagonal movement for a different
subject. (B) The joint angle plot. (C) The joint velocity plot.

between movement of the shoulder and elbow. For long periods in the
trajectory the elbow joint was inactive. A possible reason for this large
staggering in joint movement is presented in the discussion.

DISCUSSION

It is concluded that all trajectory classes can be explained by joint
interpolation in its generalized form. One question that remains to be
answered is why for some trajectories simple joint interpolation is used
while for others staggered joint interpolation is used. If staggered joint
interpolation succeeded in generating a straight line in 3B, why was it not
used to generate straight lines in 3C and 3D?

The answer lies in the observation that subjects in these experiments
almost never reversed a joint motion, either in the shoulder or in the
elbow joints. To execute a straight line motion in certain parts of the

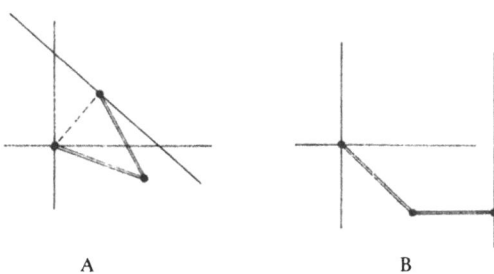

Fig. 7. (A) For a two-link manipulator following a straight line, when the endpoint reaches the normal from the shoulder to this line then elbow joint reversal occurs. (B) When the forearm is perpendicular to the straight line, shoulder joint reversal occurs.

workspace, however, joint reversal would be required. Figure 7 illustrates the situations in which joint reversal would be required. When in executing a straight line motion the endpoint reaches the intersection of the normal from the shoulder joint origin to this straight line, then elbow joint reversal would occur (Figure 7A). When the forearm is perpendicular to the straight line, shoulder joint reversal would occur (Figure 7B). Both elbow and shoulder joint reversal could occur in the same trajectory, although widely separated. Of the two, the elbow joint reversal would typically be of much larger magnitude.

In joint interpolation, it is also the case that no joint reverses itself. Simulations for the trajectories 3C and 3D are presented in Figure 8. For the vertical movements, the angle plot in Figure 8B shows that the theoretical solid line corresponding to the theoretical straight line in the Cartesian plot 8A would require a substantial amount of elbow joint reversal. The dotted lines show that no amount of staggering of elbow joint versus shoulder joint has much effect on the trajectory, since basically the elbow joint is not moving.

The joint angle plot for the inward and upward diagonal movement in Figure 8D shows that the achievement of a theoretical straight line in Figure 8C requires reversal in both the elbow and shoulder joints. The straight line in joint space generates a substantially curved motion in Cartesian space, as was seen in Figure 3D and 3H. As the staggering between the two joints is increased, the theoretical joint angle solid line is approached more closely, but it can never be reached. Evidently the best strategy would be to decouple almost completely the movement of the elbow from the movement of the shoulder. Thus although the final movement would still be curved, it would be less curved than that resulting from simple joint interpolation. This may explain why the subject in Figure 6 had a nearly decoupled joint movement. Given the restrictions on joint reversal, this subject achieved the best possible result in terms of straightening the trajectory. This was a better strategy than the simple joint interpolation used by other subjects for the same movement (Figure 3D).

Hence the reason that some trajectories are straight while others are curved is that staggered joint interpolation can often only approximate a Cartesian straight path if a joint does not reverse itself. Often simple joint interpolation is used in the cases where a straight line motion would require joint reversal (Figures 3C-D). When joint reversal would not be required to execute a straight-line motion, then staggered joint interpolation is used to achieve a very good approximation to a straight line.

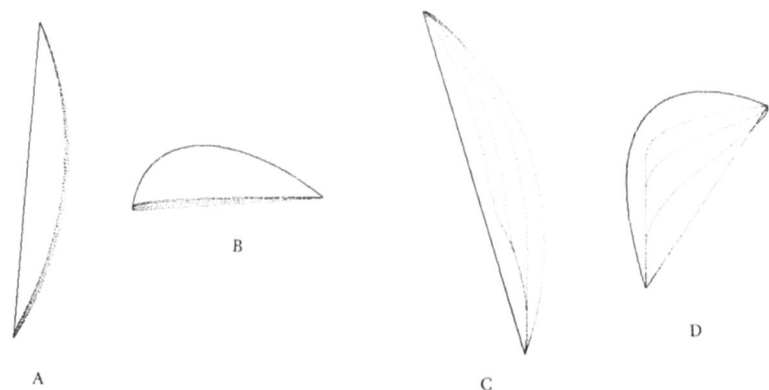

Fig. 8. (A)-(B) Simulation for the movements corresponding to Figure 3C.
The theoretical straight line in (A) (solid line) requires a
significant amount of elbow joint reversal, as seen by the solid
line in (B). Since the beginning and final elbow joint angles are
nearly the same, joint interpolation results in almost no elbow
movement, even when staggered (dotted lines in (B) and the
corresponding endpoint trajectories in (A)). (C)-(D) Simulation
for the movements corresponding to Figure 3D. The theoretical
straight line in (C) requires reversal in both shoulder and elbow
joints in (D). The more decoupled the elbow joint motion is from
the shoulder joint motion, the closer is the approximation to a
straight line.

Occasionally, subjects used staggered joint interpolation even when the end
result was a curved path for trajectories that would have required joint
reversal for a straight line. By joint decoupling, the endpoint path was
made straighter than it would have been otherwise, and represents a
judicious choice of interpolation parameters to achieve a good compromise.

The ability of a simple form of joint variable planning to generate
nearly straight trajectories in certain regions of the workspace is a
surprising result. Evidently the distinction between endpoint variable
planning and joint variable planning is not as clear cut as previously
thought. There are intermediate strategies between straight lines in joint
space and straight lines in hand space, in the present case staggered joint
interpolation, that makes a decision on planning space on the basis of the
form of the endpoint trajectory difficult. Hence these results illustrate
the dangers of arguing too closely from superficial features of data.

In generalizing the strategy of joint interpolation by adding an
adjustable parameter, one must be wary of engaging in mere curve fitting.
It is a matter of judgment whether the added reduction of the data justi-
fies the additional parameters, since the more parameters one adds to a
mathematical model, the easier it would be to fit diverse data. In the
extreme an overly parameterized joint-based planning strategy would not be
clearly distinguishable from or less complicated than an endpoint-based
planning strategy. In the present case, staggered joint interpolation
requires just one additional variable, since the time scaling is dependent
on the delay. The data reduction is an underlying explanation for both
straight and curved movements and the identification of just one planning
strategy used anywhere in the workspace.

One may speculate that staggered joint interpolation offers computational advantages to the nervous system, because an inverse kinematics

computation is obviated in intermediate parts of the trajectory. While the inverse kinematic solution must exist at the ends of the trajectory, all that would be required of the motor control system for the rest of the movement is to interpolate elbow and shoulder joints separately from start to goal and to determine an appropriate delay in relative joint onset from knowledge of these endpoints. Presumably knowledge of this delay is built up with experience, perhaps relying on feedback from vision or environmental contact constraints for learning. When indexed by the endpoints, this parameter can then be simply retrieved from motor memory. This strategy is very much simpler than an inverse kinematics computation, and would represent a clever shortcut for producing nearly straight lines. The price paid for this shortcut is a failure to produce straight trajectories in certain regions of the workspace.

It should be emphasized that these considerations are restricted to the motor tasks in the present study. The extent to which they generalize to other movement conditions is not clear. In horizontal arm movements studied with a planar pantograph, for example, joint reversal was seen in movements across the chest (Morasso, 1981). Neither were the sorts of curved movements as in the present study observed. Why there exists this difference in results between the two movement paradigms awaits further study.

Acknowledgments

This research was supported by NIH Grant AM26710 and by a grant from the Whitaker Health Sciences Fund. Personal support for SPM was provided by an NSERC Fellowship. This paper was produced using facilities of the Artificial Intelligence Lab, partially supported by DARPA contract N00014-80-C-0505.

REFERENCES

Abend, W., Bizzi, E., and Morasso, P., 1982, Human arm trajectory formation, Brain, 105:331-348.

Atkeson, C. G., and Hollerbach, J. M., 1985, Kinematic features of unrestrained vertical arm movements, J.Neuroscience, 5:2318-2330.

Bernstein, N., 1967, "The Coordination and Regulation of Movements," Pergamon Press, Oxford.

Bizzi, E., Chapple W., and Hogan, N., 1982, Mechanical properties of muscles: implications for motor control, Trends Neurosci., 5:395-398.

Bizzi, E., Accornero, N., Chapple, W., and Hogan, N., 1984, Posture control and trajectory formation during arm movement, J.Neurosci., 4:2738-2745.

Brady, J. M., 1982, Trajectory planning, in: "Robot Motion: Planning and Control," J. M. Brady, J. M. Hollerbach, T. L. Johnson, T. Lozano-Perez, and M. T. Mason, eds., MIT Press, Cambridge, Mass., p.221-243.

Flash, T., and Hogan, N., 1985, The coordination of arm movements: an experimentally confirmed mathematical model, J.Neurosci., in press.

Hildreth, E. C., and Hollerbach, J. M., 1986, The computational approach to vision and motor control, in: "Handbook of Physiology," F. Plum, ed., American Physiological Society, in press.

Hollerbach, J. M., and Atkeson, C. G., 1985, Characterization of joint-interpolated arm movements, Exp.Brain Res.Suppl., in press.

Hollerbach, J. M., and Flash, T., 1982, Dynamic interations between limb segments during planar arm movements, Biol.Cybern., 44:67-77.

Kots, Y. M., and Syrovegin, A. V., 1966, Fixed set of variants of interaction of the muscles of two joints used in the execution of simple voluntary movements, Biofizika, 11:1061-1066.

Morasso, P., 1981, Spatial control of arm movements, Exp.Brain Res., 42:223-227.

Polit, A., and Bizzi, E., 1979, Characteristics of motor programs underlying arm movements in monkeys, J.Neurophysiol., 42:183-194.

Soechting, J. F., and Lacquaniti, F., 1981, Invariant characteristics of a pointing movement in man, J.Neurosci., 1:710-720.

Soechting, J. F., Lacquaniti, F., and Terzuolo, C. A., 1985, Coordination of arm movements in three-dimensional space. Sensorimotor mapping during drawing movement, Neurosci., in press.

Soechting, J. F., and Ross, B., 1984, Psychophysical determination of coordinate representation of human arm orientation, Neurosci., 13:595-604.

KINEMATIC FORM OF LIMB AND SPEECH MOVEMENTS

D. J. Ostry, J. D. Cooke*, and K. G. Munhall**

Dept. of Psychology, McGill University, Montreal, Canada
*Dept. of Physiology, University of Western Ontario, Canada
**Haskins Laboratories, New Haven, Connecticut, USA

In this paper we ask whether there are similarities in the control of diverse motor activities by comparing the kinematic patterns of movements in two distinct behaviors: flexion and extension of the elbow and movement of the tongue dorsum in the production of speech. Our assumption is that even motor activities which are as different as limb movements and speech will share common organizational principles and those principles will be reflected in their kinematic form.

We have compared speech and limb movements by examining the form of their velocity curves. Following Nelson (1983) we have examined on a trial-to-trial basis the adherence of the kinematic patterns of movements to the relationship: $Vmax/A = c/T$, where $Vmax$ is maximum velocity, A is amplitude, T is duration, and c is a variable indicative of the form of the velocity curve. The value of c is also equal to the ratio of maximum velocity to average velocity ($\bar{V}$); that is, $c = Vmax/\bar{V}$.

If it can be shown that c remains constant for movements of different amplitude or rate then the movements share a common velocity curve (see Munhall, Ostry and Parush, 1985; Ostry and Cooke, in press). On the other hand, if the value of c is dependent on movement amplitude or duration, the geometric form of the velocity curve varies with scale changes in the movement. In this paper we demonstrate that the assumption of strict scalar equivalence of the geometric form of the velocity curve is, in general, untenable.

Kinematic measures were obtained for movements about the right elbow in response to step changes in a visual target. Subjects made movements of two different amplitudes (76° and 39°) at each of six different nominal durations (200, 300, 400, 500, 700, and 900 ms).

Movement amplitude and rate were also manipulated for tongue dorsum movements in speech. The subjects produced alternately stressed consonant-vowel sequences of the form kaká kaká ... or kokó kokó .... The sequences were produced either at a normal or a fast speech rate. In these sequences the tongue moves from a position at the palate for the production of the consonant to an open or lowered position for the production of the vowel. Both the stress and vowel manipulations produce differences in the amplitude of tongue movement, with greater amplitude, relative to a maxillary reference frame, observed for <u>a</u> than for <u>o</u> and for stressed than for un-stressed movements (see Ostry and Munhall, 1985, for review).

Figures 1 and 2 show, on a trial-to-trial basis the ratio of maximum velocity to movement amplitude plotted as a function of movement duration. Superimposed on these scatterplots is the best fit value for the variable c. The value of c was obtained by calculating the slope of the regression through the origin of Vmax/A on T. This is the value of c which would be obtained for this data if the velocity curves were members of a single scalar family.

Although the data for both articulators appear to lie on the functions predicted for constant values of c, the values of c differ in systematic ways. Values of c were, in general, higher for elbow movements than for tongue movements. The elbow movements in this study were discrete movements; the arm started and ended at rest. In contrast, the tongue dorsum movement was essentially cyclical. For comparison purposes, the value of c corresponding to the minimum jerk trajectory in discrete movements is

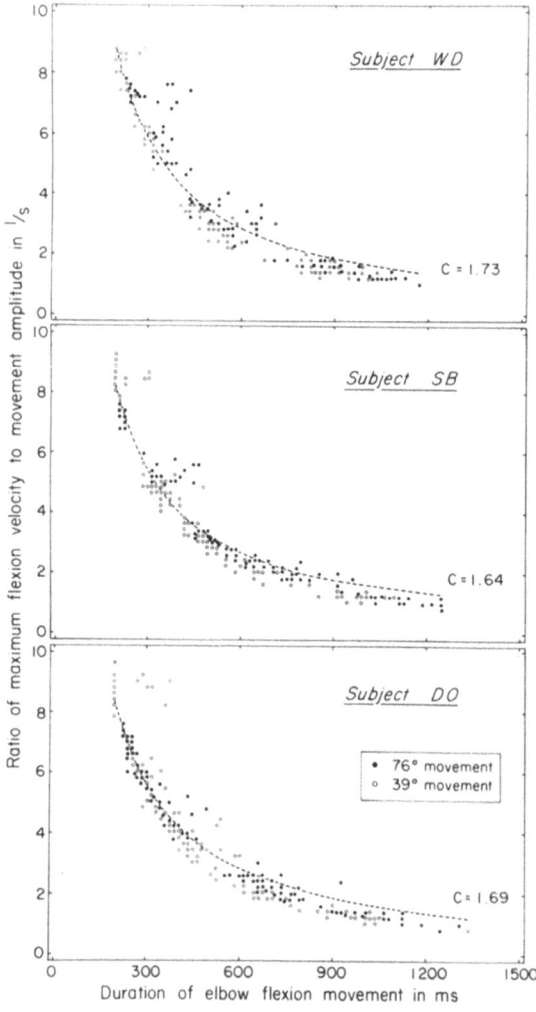

Fig. 1.   Ratio of maximum velocity to movement amplitude for elbow flexion movements plotted as a function of movement duration.

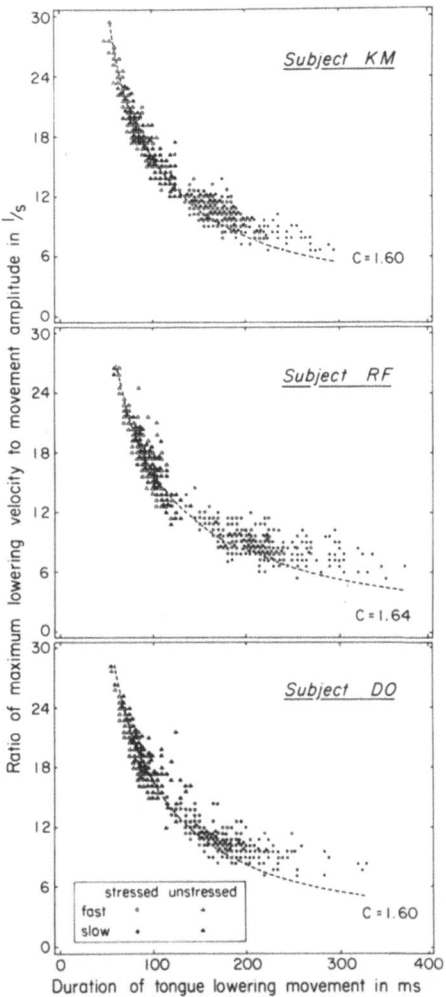

Fig. 2. Ratio of maximum velocity to movement amplitude for tongue dorsum lowering movements plotted as a function of movement duration.

1.88 (Hogan, 1984); for cyclical movements, the value of c, again for the minimum jerk trajectory, is 1.56 (Nelson, 1983).

Values of c, for both the tongue dorsum and the elbow also varied in a systematic way with differences in movement duration. In Figure 3, the average values for c for elbow and tongue movements have been computed for each experimental condition. In elbow movements, it can be seen that the values of c decrease as movements increase in duration. In contrast, for tongue movements, c increases as a function of duration. The variation in c indicates that, in this study, the velocity curves of arm and tongue movements do not form geometrically equivalent families.

For limb movements, the regression of c on T, shown in Figure 3, has the form: c = 1.94 - 0.69T, where T is movement time in seconds. For tongue movements, the regression of c on T gives: c = 1.39 + 2.40T, again with T in seconds. In both cases, the slopes differ reliably from zero (p < 0.001).

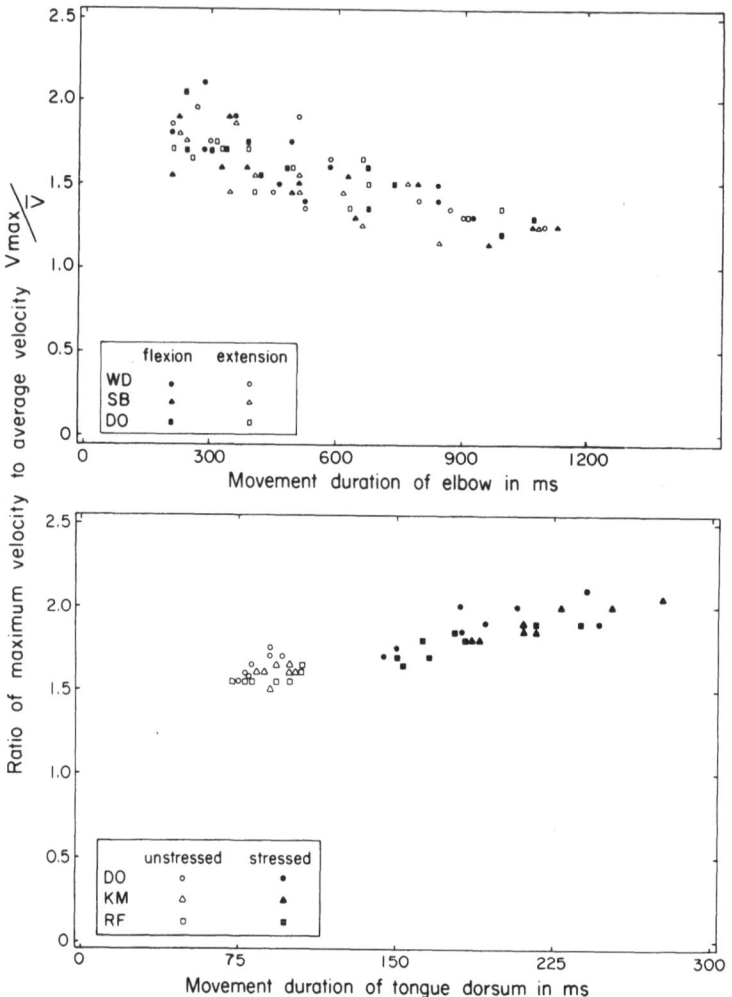

Fig. 3. Average values of c as a function of movement duration for both elbow and tongue dorsum movements.

The departures from geometrical equivalence of the velocity curves of both arm and tongue movements can be simulated by changing the damping ratio in a lumped parameter second order model of the articulator. Geometrical equivalence of velocity curves is observed in simulations only when the damping ratio is constant. As the damping ratio is decreased, the value of c increases.

In conclusion, we find for both speech and limb movements that the form of the velocity curve varies systematically with changes in movement duration. These variations can be simulated by varying the damping ratio of the limb. The nervous system presumably exploits these dynamical characteristics of articulators in the production of various kinds of voluntary movement ranging from simple reaching movements to linguistic gestures.

Acknowledgements

This research was supported by grants from NSERC (Canada), MRC (Canada), FCAR (Quebec) and an NINCDS program project grant NS-13617 (US).

REFERENCES

Hogan, N., 1984, An organizing principle for a class of voluntary movements, J.Neurosci., 4:2745-2754.

Munhall, K. G., Ostry, D. J., and Parush, A., 1985, Characteristics of velocity profiles of speech movements, J.Experim.Psychol:Human Perception & Performance, 11:457-474.

Nelson, W. L., 1983, Physical principles for economies of skilled movements, Biol.Cybernetics, 46:135-147.

Ostry, D. J., and Cooke, J. D., in press, Kinematic characteristics of speech and limb movements, in: "Motor and Sensory Processes of Language", E. Keller and M. Gopnik, eds., Lawrence Erlbaum Associates.

Ostry, D. J., and Munhall, K. G., 1985, Control of rate and duration of speech movements, J.Acoustical Soc.of Amer., 77:640-648.

SYNERGETICS AT MOTONEURON LEVEL

(Diffuse projection systems, instant field and behavior of the pool)

St. Baykushev

Professor of Neurology
Higher Medical Institute I. P. Pavlov
Plovdiv, Bulgaria

Recently Hermann Haken (1983; 1984) formulated the aims of a new, interdisciplinary, scientific direction – Synergetics: phenomena of self-organization in physics, chemistry, and biology.

Sharing Hacken's opinion that synergetics could give some new impulses to brain research, this description and analysis of brain function in terms of synergetics was made. It could give rise, however, to some notions of general importance too (especially in the line function-structure, e.g., how the structure was born).

What is the mechanism of the synergies in the CNS and the effectors? Ashby (1960) described the nervous system or a part of it as an arbitrary selected set of variables. The state of the system at a given instant is the set of numerical values which the variables have at this instant and the line of behavior is specified by a succession of states and the time intervals between them. The variables in the system are essential (which are to be maintained in some physiological limits) and supplementary (which variations serve to maintain the essential in the limits). The variables within the system and those out of the system do not differ in their intrinsic physical nature. They are connected, except for that particular instant, when the connection is at a zero point. The variables not included in the system play the role of parameters for the arbitrary selected system. The effective parameters are innumerable but certain ones may be particularly important. Changes of value of significant (or order) parameters change the field of the system, and the system stability depends upon its field. So long as a significant parameter is constant the system with changing variables may display a change of state. A change of the value of a significant effective parameter changes the line of behavior.

Starting from this description let us take the most simple example of a homogeneous final population of neurons, such as in a primitive multicellular organism with uniform mode of movement, or as in an anterior horn motoneuron pool, with uniform action. The synergy will take place here in the action of the separate elements of the population which are "all or not" elements and may act or not act. (The readiness to action is, however, a discrete function.) Every element y of this population M(motoneurons) is a function of the action of some or of the entire elements of a second subpopulation X_i, i.e.,

$$y = F(X_i); \quad X_i = \{X_i\}; \quad X < A,$$

and this subpopulation X is included in a greater population A (different kinds of afferentation). The dependence is of probability kind (Chernish and Napalkov, 1964).

Every element of the X-population (afferent neurons) ends on a number of y-elements, i.e., has got a diffuse projection, and so is the system as a whole.

The simplicity is only a superficial one. The population of motoneurons and every single element undergo the influence of many converging influences, which are making the instant field and determine the number of active and fringe motoneurons and the behavior of the population. This situation is analyzed in another work (Baykushev, 1970).

Let us go further to the analysis of a withdrawal reflex in the legs (normal as well as pathological) arising on the ground of a sustained posture. The situation here is more complicated as many more muscle groups of synergists and antagonists are involved at different joint levels (resp. different spinal segment levels), e.g., the synergy is spread over many populations of motoneurons.

Because a complex movement must be realized at many of the extremity's joints, not only a positive (excitatory) synergic involvement of different degree in all of the many different motoneuron populations, but also an inhibition arises simultaneously in some other antagonist motoneuron population. In respect to the general action, this is a synergic coinnervation (because it enables the action), but it is negative (inhibitory). The innervation is diffuse but structuralized, i.e., has got a pattern.

Nevertheless, the system could be regarded in the same way as above, taking now as variables the homogeneous motoneuron pools and as significant parameters the afferents, i.e., as a diffuse and structuralized system.

This example shows how the diffuse projections determine the phase field of a neuronal system.

Some different states of such a system could be described when a sustained contraction is programed and carried out. If the effective (or order) parameters are at a zero point the system is steady at a state of rest. This is normally a very rare case (in deep sleep and relaxation of the leg for example).

If (a) the postural efferent innervation is standing and the proprioceptive afferentation is varying in some narrow limits the field and respectively the system is steady. The variables could undergo changes but the changes end in a point (or rather circle) of balance and the system tends to maintain a steady state. This is a maintained position of the leg.

If (b) one of the order parameters (afferentation by a painful stimulation of the foot) is changed, the line of behavior of the system is changed and the variable tends to reach some border declination. In the real body space scheme this is the triple flexion of the leg. Ceasing the stimulation, e.g., changing of the order parameters or the pattern of the diffuse innervation, leads to the formation of a new phase-field resp. a new stage of state.

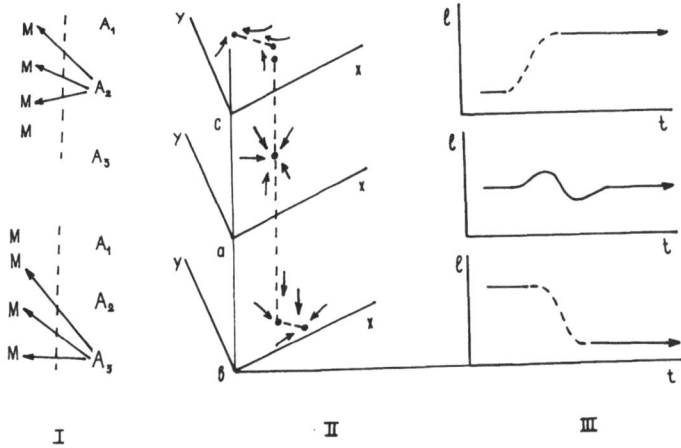

I   II   III

Fig. 1. A balance contraction of flexors subserving a sustained posture and different mode of programing. (I) afferent neuron populations (A) as effective parameters; motoneuron populations (M), as important variables. A_1 – proprioceptive afferentation; A_2 – exteroceptive painful afferentation from the front of the hip; A_3 – as the latter, from the foot. (II) point of equilibrium in a two-dimensional (x, y) scale. (III) line of equilibrium in a scale "length of muscle/time" (l, t). An attempt is made to present how the diffuse projection systems determine the phase-field and respectively the behavior of the motoneuron populations during equilibrium (a), flexor (b) and extensor (c) withdrawal reflexes of the leg.

Vice versa (c), the painful afferent inflow from the frontal surface of the hip, as an order parameter, leads to reverse sign (direction) of declination for the same variable (length of flexors) but for positive declination of other (reciprocal) variables (length of extensors). Together this forms a row of stage-states of a system with different phase-fields. The action is lavin-like in both latter examples and ceases in an end position.

This is a new higher degree of development of the diffuse projection systems as a basis of the synergies.

Anatomically and functionally better developed diffuse projection systems are for example the reticulo-spinal influences of the reticular formation and the COEP (cortical originating extrapyramidal) system. The first is the basis of the so-called static synergies (global synkineses) and the second of some kinetic synergies (mirror synkineses of different type in leg and arm). These two types of synergy (Baykushev, 1982; 1984) differ mainly in respect to their reciprocal organization.

This last shows the different degree of organization, not only in respect to neuronal structures, but also as a space-time distribution, i.e., as a pattern. At last, this leads in evolution and corticalization to a transition from diffuse to more or less specific superposed systems, with more correct and restricted areas of influence.

One could see, however, that even when a specific system is involved in action (for example, an intended movement to take a glass of water), it is supplemented with programed foregoing and simultaneous synergies (ensuring that the man will take the glass and not instead fall on his face to the ground, because of changing body weight center and loss of equilibrium).

A learned, conditioned motor act at the very beginning is displayed at the specific systems and accompanied with activity of diffuse ones. But even the most attentive initial performance is one with a wide (and later unnecessary) range of irradiation. Here again the reaction and its parts go the same way as a primitive and pure structured action.

The perfection of the synergies in evolution were driven from the mere projection of influences to structural systems and a space-time pattern, and from diffuse to more or less specific but wide spread systems.

The same goes for the development and perfection of the sensory and other nervous functions. The psychic functions are not excluded either: the connection between emotions and the vegetative class of events is a matter of diffuse projection at the level diencephalon hypophysis (including hormon-humoral), reticular, and limbic systems. These systems are at the same time diffuse and specific ones.

The following outlines the synergetics at motor neuron level:

(1) the basis of synergies are the diffuse projection systems;
(2) the evolution as well as the elaboration of a synergic action goes from the diffuse projection to a reciprocal structuralization (anatomical or functional) with presentation of positive as well as negative components;
(3) the pattern of the action is different at the same level (in the same group of subunits) as far as some influences act as effective parameters of the system and change the field, resp. the behavior of the system;
(4) the integrity of action and literally the integrity of organisms is secured by the synergies;
(5) this underlines the universal importance of the diffuse projection systems; and
(6) the synergies subserve the formation of pattern and structure and their preservation.

REFERENCES

Ashby, W. R., 1960, "Design of a Brain", Chapman and Hall, London.
Baykushev, St., 1970, Desynchronization of the excitatory process in the α-motoneurons and its role for the performance of motor actions, Folia Medica, XII,II:95-107.
Baykushev, St., 1977, The role of the synergies and the creation of their basis feedback in the processes of restoration of movements after cerebral vascular accidents, Dissert.Med.Sci., Plovdiv (Bulgarian, summary in English).
Baykushev, St., 1983, EMG analysis of mirror synkinesias' role in the motor re-education of patients with central paralyses. Nerve und Muscle Symposium, Greifswaldt, 1982, Z.Ernst-Mortiz-Arndt-Universität, Greifswaldt, 32,3:46-50.
Baykushev, St., 1984, Kinetic and static synergies and their role in the motor re-education after cerebral stroke, Electromyogr.Clin. Neurophysiol., 24:81-90.
Chernish, V. I., and Napalkov, A. V., 1964, Mathematical apparatus of biological cybernetics, Moskva, Medizina (in Russian).
Haken, H., 1983, "Synergetik", Eine Einführung, Springer.
Haken, H., 1984, Synergetik - Selbstorganisationsvorgänge in Physik, Chemie und Biologie, Mitteilungen, A.v. Humboldt-Stiftung, März, 43:12-23.

INDEX

Arm
  forward elevation, 111–116
  loading, muscle recruitment
        changes due to, 112, 114
  movement kinematics, joint
        interpolation, 197–207
Axons
  recurrent inhibitory postsynaptic
        potentials of single motor,
        20
  stimulation of single motor, 20

Bereitschaftspotential, 93, 99

Electrodes
  floating, freely moving cats, 156,
        160
  surface selective branched EMG, 7,
        8

Golgi receptors, 63–66

Hypotonia, 51, 52

Locomotion
  Ia afferents antidromic discharges
        during, 165–169
  single motor units firing during,
        16, 17
  speed independent invariants model
        of, 177
  ventral spinocerebellar tract
        neurons activity during,
        155–158

Methods
  antiorthostatic bedrest, 149
  dry immersion, 149
  induced body oscillations, 129,
        130
  single motor axon stimulation, 19,
        20
  single motor units recording, 13
  single muscle fiber micro-
        chemistry, 23
  single ventral root axons
        recording, 160

Methods (continued)
  spike-triggered averaging, 156,
        157, 160
  time series analysis, 145–147
  time varying identification, 190
  vestibular galvanic stimulation,
        141, 142
Models
  of locomotion, 177
  one joint motor control, 183–186
Motoneurons
  α, activity during walking, 159–163
  α, activity during flexor reflexes,
        159–163
  hypoglossal, paleocerebellar
        modulation of, 69–73
  synergetics at the level of,
        215–218
Motor control
  equilibrium point hypothesis, 184
  cortex lesions, task performance,
        80–84
  one joint model, 183–186
  support unloading effect on 149–152
  system identification: time varying
        techniques, 189–194
  of tongue muscle, transcerebellar
        loop, 69
Motor units
  fatiguability vs. single fiber
        microchemistry, 23
  firing pattern, support unloading,
        150
  single, Ia afferents stimulation,
        60
  single, firing pattern of, 7–9
  single, m. extensor digitorum
        brevis, 13
  single, m. interosseus dorsalis I,
        7
  single, low and high threshold, 13
Movements
  higher disturbances in monkey,
        79–84
  hippocampal EEG during, 75–78
  kinematics of limb and speech,
        209–212

Movements (continued)
role of premotor cortex, 84
staggered joint interpolation
strategy, 197
vestibulomotor response
facilitation due to
voluntary, 141–143
Movements related brain potentials
isometric voluntary contraction,
93–97
fatiguing hand contractions,
99–102
Muscle
"catch-like" phenomenon, 4
contraction, H-reflex, 61
contraction, postural and phasic
modes of, 5
force, rising factors of, 10
force sensation due to co-
contraction, 105–108
recruitment in arm movement,
111–116
stiffness, hypotonia, 54
stiffness, posture control, 132
Muscle fibers
fatigue resistance and metabolic
capacity dissociation, 25
single, microchemistry, 23

Neurons
dentate, reaction time tasks,
87–90
of ventral spinocerebellar tract,
locomotion, 155–158

Posture
afferent control of, 135–139
bulbar reticular unit activity
during, 199–125
striatal control of, 123–126
time series analysis of, 145–148
visual feedback control of,
129–132

Reflexes
cutaneous, in children, 31–34
cutaneous, ontogenetic stages, 34
flexor, motoneurons activity
during, 159–163
H-, antiorthostatic bedrest, 151,
152
H-, presynaptic inhibition, 59–62
M2-A long latency spinal, 37
stretch, changes due to hypotonia,
51–58
stretch, hemiplegics patients, 47
stretch, inhibition during gait,
135, 136
stretch, ischemic nerve block, 45
stretch, posture control, 132
stretch, skin afferents
stimulation, 37–41, 46
stretch, vibration, 43, 44
T-, antiorthostatic bedrest, 151,
152

Step cycle
perturbations, forelimb responses,
171–174
single motor activity during, 16,
17
stretch reflex during, 136

Task
performance, support unloading, 150
simple reaction time-, dentate
neurons, 87–90
visual motor conditional-, cortex
lesions, 81
visual non motor conditional-,
cortex lesions, 81
Tetanus
phases of unfused, 4